SOFT TISSUE AND BONE PATHOLOGY

PATHOLOGY

A Question and Answer Based Review

SOFT TISSUE AND BONE PATHOLOGY

A Question and Answer Based Review

Agedi Boto MD PhD
Clinical Fellow
Yale-New Haven Hospital
Connecticut, USA

Jose Costa MD
Professor
Pathology and Medicine (Oncology)
Professor
Orthopedics and Rehabilitation
Yale University School of Medicine
Connecticut, USA

JAYPEE *The Health Sciences Publisher*
Philadelphia | New Delhi | London | Panama

Jaypee Brothers Medical Publishers (P) Ltd

Headquarters

Jaypee Brothers Medical Publishers (P) Ltd
4838/24, Ansari Road, Daryaganj
New Delhi 110 002, India
Phone: +91-11-43574357
Fax: +91-11-43574314
Email: jaypee@jaypeebrothers.com

Overseas Offices

J.P. Medical Ltd
83, Victoria Street, London
SW1H 0HW (UK)
Phone: +44 20 3170 8910
Fax: +44 (0)20 3008 6180
Email: info@jpmedpub.com

Jaypee-Highlights Medical Publishers Inc
City of Knowledge, Bld. 235, 2nd Floor, Clayton
Panama City, Panama
Phone: +1 507-301-0496
Fax: +1 507-301-0499
Email: cservice@jphmedical.com

Jaypee Medical Inc
325 Chestnut Street
Suite 412, Philadelphia, PA 19106, USA
Phone: +1 267-519-9789
Email: support@jpmedus.com

Jaypee Brothers Medical Publishers (P) Ltd
17/1-B Babar Road, Block-B, Shaymali
Mohammadpur, Dhaka-1207
Bangladesh
Mobile: +08801912003485
Email: jaypeedhaka@gmail.com

Jaypee Brothers Medical Publishers (P) Ltd
Bhotahity, Kathmandu, Nepal
Phone +977-9741283608
Email: kathmandu@jaypeebrothers.com

Website: www.jaypeebrothers.com
Website: www.jaypeedigital.com

Soft Tissue and Bone Pathology: A Question and Answer Based Review

First Edition: **2017**

ISBN 978-93-86056-02-3

Printed at Sanat Printers

Dedication

This learning tool is dedicated to the house-staff in pathology to help them succeed in caring for their patients.

Preface

This book is designed to be a study tool for trainees in pathology to exercise and gauge their knowledge about the pathology of tumors and tumor-like conditions occurring in the musculoskeletal system and somatic soft tissues. Trainees in orthopedic surgery and musculoskeletal radiology may also find it useful.

We aim to provide a series of challenges to test the reader and stimulate further learning and expertise in what is seen by many as a challenging diagnostic terrain. This book is not, therefore, a systematic presentation of entities, their features, and differential diagnosis. There are already in print excellent sections on soft tissue and bone pathology in general surgical pathology texts, as well as a number of specialized treatises, where trainees can find comprehensive and systematic sources of such information.

As a consequence of our major aim, we present the material under a series of differential diagnostic scenarios that should stimulate the reader to follow or create diagnostic algorithms based on the information contained in the major textbooks and their personal experience. Many of the required responses to the questions do not consist simply of 'what it is', but require epidemiological clinical knowledge and an awareness of molecular descriptors of the disease, because the molecular diagnostic field promises ultimate precision in the diagnosis of many entities.

The pictures presented should be regarded as prompts only, as it would be unrealistic to make an accurate diagnostic interpretation from a single field. Limitations in scope have forced a selection and sampling of entities that is far from exhaustive. Completeness has been sacrificed to the reiteration of some entities that we believe merit emphasis. We also chose to be brief, encouraging the reader to work through the book more than once, as repetition is important for learning.

The case selections and any errors in this book are the sole responsibility of the authors.

Agedi Boto MD PhD
Jose Costa MD

Acknowledgments

We are indebted to our Yale Sarcoma Program colleagues that make the delivery of high-quality care to patients with lesions of the musculoskeletal system possible. We are also grateful for the support and help from the technical staff and the graphics unit of the Department of Pathology at the Yale University School of Medicine and Yale-New Haven Hospital, Connecticut, USA. This book would not have been possible without the thorough editing and proofreading by the editorial staff of Jaypee Brothers Medical Publishers (P) Ltd. Lastly, we would like to thank our colleagues, who characterized and studied these lesions initially, and whose work fills these pages. Their contributions have and will continue to improve the diagnostic accuracy of the pathologists.

We would like to thank Mr Jitendar P Vij (Group Chairman), Mr Ankit Vij (Group President), Ms Chetna Malhotra Vohra (Associate Director), Mr Umar Rashid (Development Editor), and the production team of Jaypee Brothers Medical Publishers (P) Ltd, New Delhi, India.

Contents

1. Monotonous Spindle Cell Lesions: Benign, Malignant and Pseudosarcomatous   1–32

2. Pleomorphic Lesions   33–51

3. Benign Entities   52–61

4. Lesions with a Prominent Vascular Component   62–76

5. Lesions with a Prominent Myxoid Component   77–88

6. Lesions with Epithelioid Cells or Abundant Vacuolated/Amphophilic/Eosinophilic Cytoplasm   89–106

7. Lytic and Cystic Lesions of Bones and Joints   107–116

8. Small Round Blue Cell Tumors   117–126

9. Joint and Bone Lesions with Giant Cells   127–132

10. Lesions Forming Bone and Cartilage   133–151

Index   153–154

CHAPTER 1

Monotonous Spindle Cell Lesions:
Benign, Malignant and Pseudosarcomatous

1. **A 30-year-old patient with HIV and diffuse mesenteric lymphadenopathy has an excisional biopsy of what appears to be a lymph node. Histology from the excision is shown to the right and an EBER stain is shown in the inset. Desmin and SMA stains are positive. What is the correct diagnosis?**
   (a) Leiomyoma
   (b) GIST
   (c) EBV-associated smooth muscle tumor
   (d) Schwannoma
   (e) Leiomyosarcoma

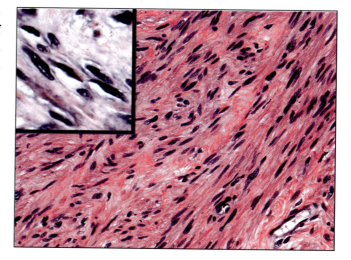

2. **A 50-year-old HIV positive patient has the submental mass depicted to the right and a brain mass. The clinical suspicion is lymphoma. What is the correct diagnosis?**
   (a) Patch-stage Kaposi sarcoma
   (b) Kaposiform hemangioendothelioma
   (c) Nodular Kaposi sarcoma
   (d) Spindle cell angiosarcoma
   (e) Granulomatous lymph node

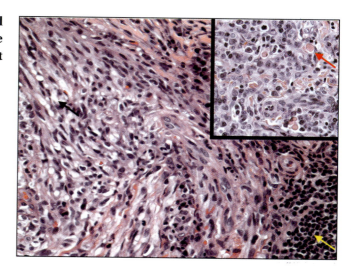

3. **An 11-year-old boy has a right cheek mass that stains positive for SMA and negatively for CD34 and desmin. What is the correct diagnosis?**
   (a) Leiomyoma
   (b) Granulomatous inflammation
   (c) Epithelioid sarcoma
   (d) Granuloma annulare
   (e) Myofibroma

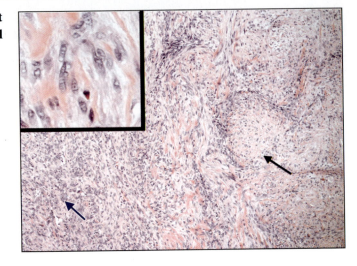

4. **A 60-year-old female has a 4.9 cm heterogeneously enhancing solid mass along the left pelvic sidewall, impinging on the obturator fossa. Histology form the lesion is shown to the right. What is the correct diagnosis?**
   (a) Fibromatosis
   (b) Ancient schwannoma
   (c) Neurofibroma
   (d) Plexiform neurofibroma
   (e) Malignant peripheral nerve sheath tumor

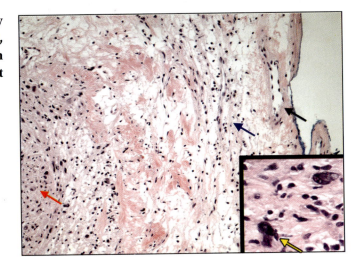

5. **The infiltrative lesion depicted in this image most likely stains positively for which of the following stains?**
   (a) AE1/AE3
   (b) Beta-catenin
   (c) CD34
   (d) Desmin
   (e) S-100

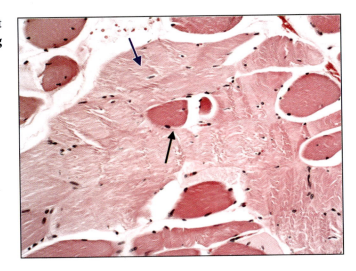

6. **A 1-year-old male has a 0.6 cm mass at the distal aspect of the fourth left phalanx. What is the correct diagnosis?**
   (a) Infantile digital fibroma
   (b) Inclusion body fibromatosis
   (c) Dupuytren's contracture
   (d) Desmoid fibromatosis
   (e) Infantile desmoid fibromatosis

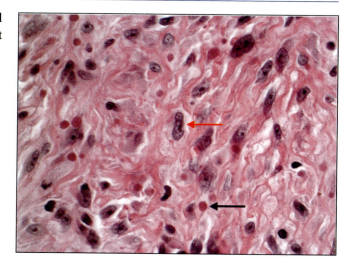

7. **A 46-year-old man has a 6 cm retroperitoneal mass. What is the correct diagnosis?**
   (a) Neuroblastoma
   (b) Ganglioneuroblastoma
   (c) Ganglioneuroma
   (d) Malignant melanoma
   (e) Plasma cell neoplasm

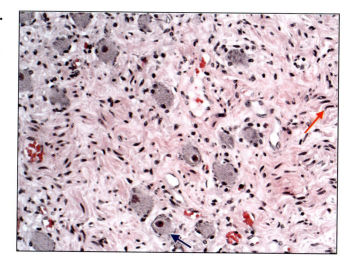

8. **A 64-year-old woman has a well-circumscribed 2.6 cm left temporal region mass fixed to but not invading bone. She has a clinical history of a fever with an elevated ESR. The tumor cells stain positively for ALK. What is the correct diagnosis?**
   (a) Inflammatory pleomorphic undifferentiated sarcoma
   (b) Inflammatory myofibroblastic tumor
   (c) Myxoinflammatory fibroblastic sarcoma
   (d) Hodgkin lymphoma
   (e) Anaplastic large cell lymphoma

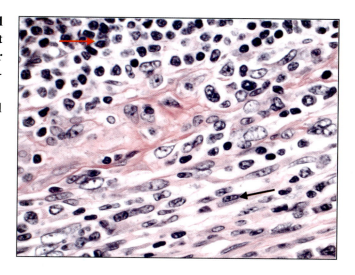

9. **A 50-year-old female has a left tibial mass. Imaging is nondiagnostic. What is the correct diagnosis?**
   (a) Nodular fasciitis
   (b) Ischemic fasciitis
   (c) Fibromatosis
   (d) Low grade fibromyxoid sarcoma
   (e) Myofibromatosis

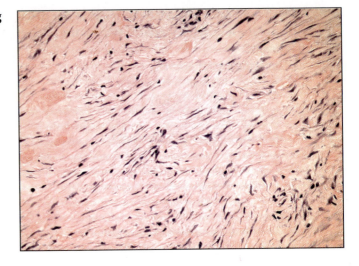

10. **A 50-year-old female has a large enhancing mass in the superficial left popliteal fossa. The lesion recurred but never metastasized. What is the correct diagnosis?**
    (a) Fibrosarcoma
    (b) Schwannoma
    (c) Desmoid fibromatosis
    (d) Fibrolipoma
    (e) Myofibroma

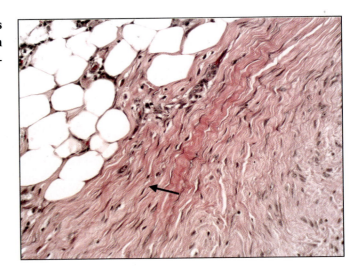

11. **A 58-year-old female has a history of facial numbness. Imaging shows a heterogeneously enhancing mass in the left temporal fossa extending to the middle cranial fossa. This lesion went on to recur and metastasize to the lungs. Smooth muscle actin and desmin are positive. H-caldesmon is negative. What is the correct diagnosis?**
    (a) Fibrosarcoma
    (b) Osteosarcoma
    (c) Fibrous dysplasia
    (d) Low grade myofibroblastic sarcoma
    (e) Leiomyosarcoma

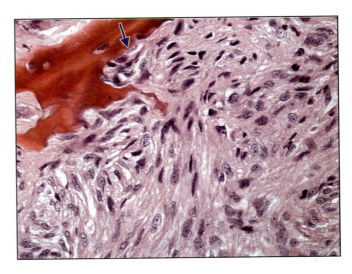

12. **A 12-year-old female had left lower leg pain for 2 days without trauma. X-rays demonstrate a locally destructive proximal metaphyseal fibular lesion. What is the correct diagnosis?**

  (a) Nonossifying fibroma
  (b) Low grade fibrosarcoma
  (c) Desmoplastic fibroma
  (d) Well-differentiated intramedullary osteosarcoma
  (e) Fibromatosis

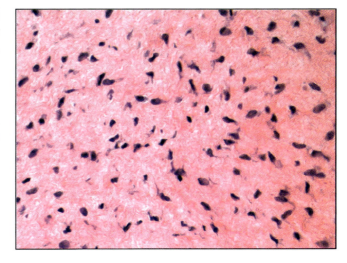

13. **A 25-year-old female has a well-circumscribed 3 cm soft tissue mass of the right lateral thigh. What is the correct diagnosis?**

  (a) Schwannoma
  (b) Neurofibroma
  (c) Dermatofibroma
  (d) Superficial angiomyxoma
  (e) Desmoplastic fibroblastoma

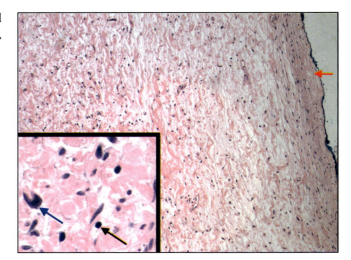

14. **Which of the following stains is likely to strongly and diffusely stain the spindled cells depicted in this excision of a well-circumscribed soft tissue nodule?**

  (a) S-100
  (b) CD34
  (c) Factor XIIIA
  (d) Actin
  (e) Desmin

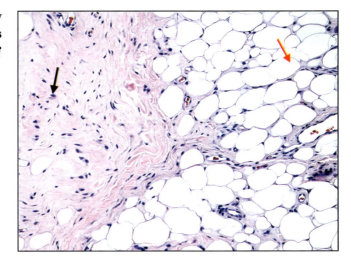

15. **A 78-year-old female has a slow growing firm left breast nodule. Tumor cells stain positively for CD34. What is the correct diagnosis?**
    (a) Dermatofibroma
    (b) Myofibroblastoma
    (c) Dermatofibrosarcoma protuberans
    (d) Spindle cell lipoma
    (e) Angiomyofibroblastoma

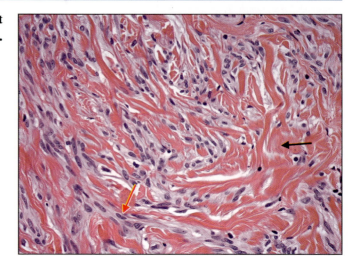

16. **A 6-year-old girl has multiple tumors on the thumb, index finger, and mouth none of which exhibit a periosteal reaction on imaging. She also complains that she can not relax her joints sometimes. What is the correct diagnosis?**
    (a) Neurothekeoma
    (b) Myxoid chondrosarcoma
    (c) Juvenile hyaline fibromatosis
    (d) Myxofibrosarcoma
    (e) Myxoma

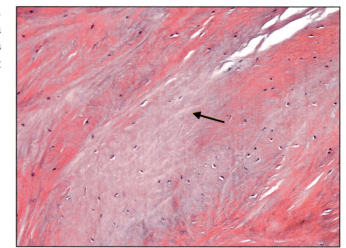

17. **A 10-year-old boy has a right anterior superior iliac spine lesion. What is the correct diagnosis?**
    (a) Fibromatosis
    (b) Chondroma
    (c) Calcifying aponeurotic fibroma
    (d) Calciphylaxis
    (e) Chondrosarcoma with dystrophic calcifications

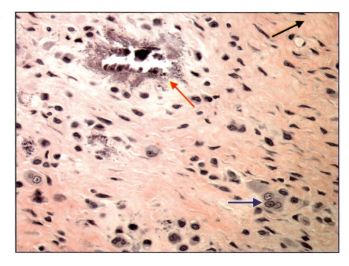

18. **A 12-year-old has a 14 cm irregular solid mass attached to the mid pole of the left kidney and displacing the tail of the pancreas. The lesion stains for S-100. What is the correct diagnosis?**
    (a) Wilm's tumor
    (b) Neuroblastoma
    (c) GIST
    (d) Neurofibroma
    (e) Cellular schwannoma

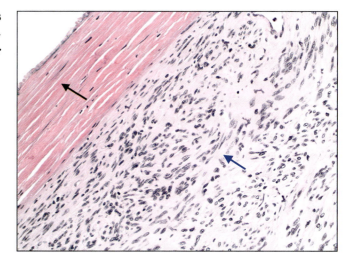

19. **A 59-year-old male has a superficial nodule in the skin overlying his right leg. What is the correct diagnosis?**
    (a) Dermatofibroma
    (b) DFSP
    (c) Neurothekeoma
    (d) Neurofibroma
    (e) Scar

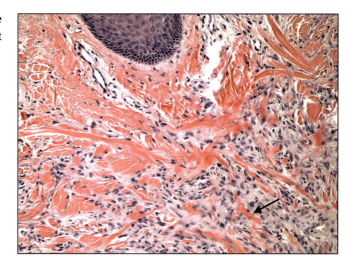

20. **A 20-year-old man has a 9 cm retroperitoneal mass. What do the eosinophilic cells marked by the blue arrow stain positively for?**
    (a) CD34
    (b) CD99
    (c) Desmin
    (d) S-100
    (e) No markers

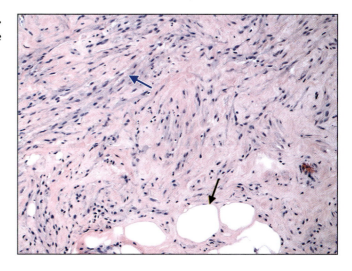

21. A 10-year-old girl has a 4.2 cm mass of her right face. Histology from the lesion is shown to the right. What clinical syndrome is she most likely afflicted with?

   (a) NF2

   (b) NF1

   (c) Tuberous sclerosis

   (d) Sturge-Weber syndrome

   (e) Mafucci syndrome

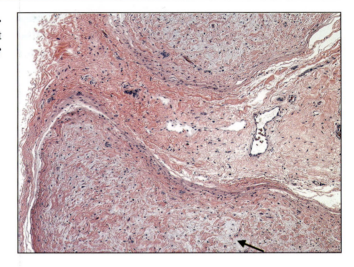

22. A 23-year-old man has a posterior thoracic wall tumor. Histology from the lesion is depicted to the right. What clinical syndrome is this tumor closely associated with?

   (a) NF1

   (b) NF2

   (c) Carney complex

   (d) Carney triad

   (e) Tuberous sclerosis

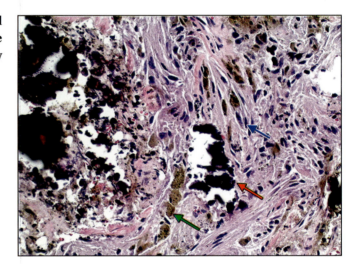

23. This 1 cm lesion on the finger of a 1-year-old displays bright eosinophilic inclusions on high power. Which of the following stains is most likely to be negative in lesional cells?

   (a) Smooth muscle actin

   (b) Desmin

   (c) Nuclear beta-catenin

   (d) CD99

   (e) CD117

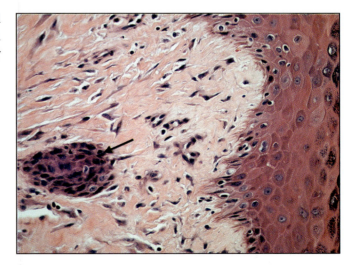

24. **A 43-year-old man has a left middle finger phalangeal amputation for necrotizing fasciitis. Now there is a painful bulb at the amputation stump. Histology from the bulb is shown to the right. What is the correct diagnosis?**
    (a) Neurofibroma
    (b) Traumatic neuroma
    (c) Schwannoma
    (d) Leiomyoma
    (e) Mucosal neuroma

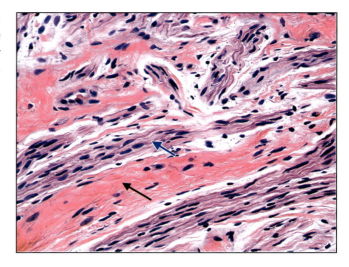

25. **A 10-year-old girl has a well-circumscribed 2.1 cm right dorsal wrist mass that stains positively for S-100 and is shown to the right. What is the correct diagnosis?**
    (a) Dermatofibroma
    (b) Neurofibroma
    (c) Perineurioma
    (d) DFSP
    (e) Schwannoma

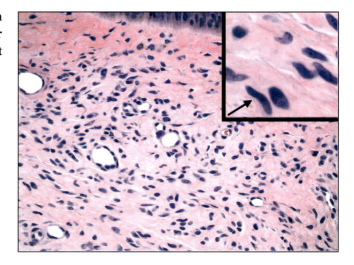

26. **A 4-month-old has what appears to be a congenital band in the left soleus with fatty infiltration beginning 3.5 cm below the knee joint. 8 cm below the joint line there is another band. Gastrocnemius atrophy is identified. What is the correct diagnosis?**
    (a) Myofibroma
    (b) Myofibromatosis
    (c) Congenital fibrosarcoma
    (d) Hemangiopericytoma
    (e) Fibrous hamartoma of infancy

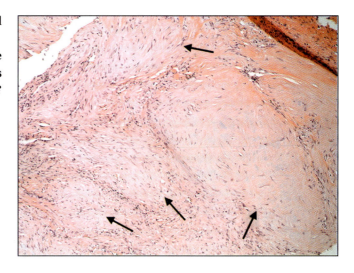

27. Which stain is used to distinguish this benign tumor from dermatofibrosarcoma protuberans (DFSP)?

(a) S-100

(b) Desmin

(c) CD34

(d) Pancytokeratin

(e) Vimentin

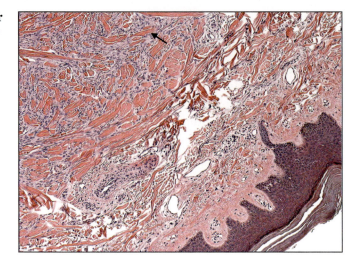

28. A 41-year-old man had a fall on ice 5 months ago. His shoulder is still bothering him; an X-ray shows a deltoid mass but no fracture. A biopsy of the mass is shown to the right. What is the correct diagnosis?

(a) Ganglioneuroma

(b) Ganglioneuroblastoma

(c) Metastatic signet ring cell carcinoma

(d) Proliferative myositis

(e) Nodular fasciitis

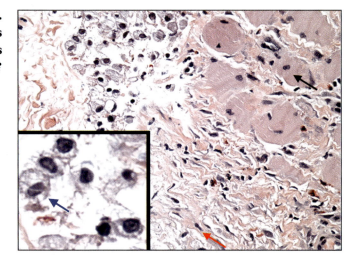

29. A 15-month-old has a 2.5 mm dermally-anchored mass in the left posterior neck. Some regions stain positively for alcian blue. What is the correct diagnosis?

(a) Gardner fibroma

(b) Nuchal type fibroma

(c) Fibrous hamartoma of infancy

(d) Myofibroma

(e) Granuloma annulare

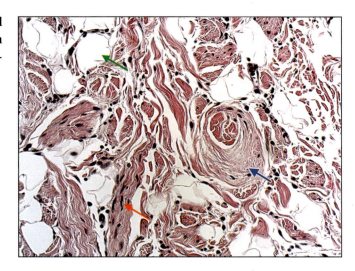

30. A 70-year-old man has problems straightening his ring finger. An excision from a scar-like firm area is depicted. What is the most specific correct diagnosis?

(a) Fibromatosis
(b) Dupuytren's contracture
(c) Myofibromatosis
(d) Low grade fibromyxoid sarcoma
(e) Low grade myofibroblastic sarcoma

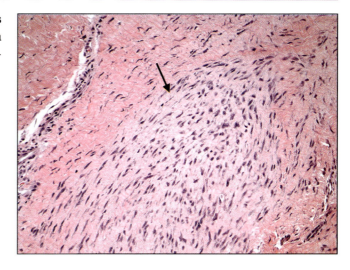

31. A 49-year-old female has a painless well-circumscribed left labia minora lesion. Shown to the right is a high power view of the exclusively dermal lesion. What is the correct diagnosis?

(a) Cellular angiofibroma
(b) Angiomyxoma
(c) Lobular capillary hemangioma
(d) Angiomyofibroblastoma
(e) Dermatofibroma

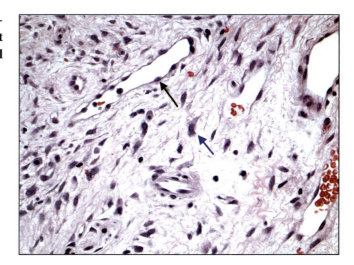

32. What chromosomal changes are typically associated with the lesion depicted to the right?

(a) Loss of 16q, 13q
(b) Gain of 16q, 13q
(c) Ring chromosomes
(d) Giant marker chromosomes
(e) Complex multifocal cytogenetic changes

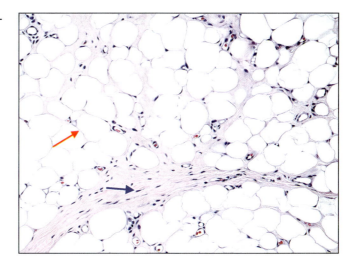

33. A 45-year-old man has a 2 cm nasal mass. What stain will most likely highlight the neoplastic cells?
    (a) Vimentin
    (b) Desmin
    (c) Actin
    (d) Keratin
    (e) CD34

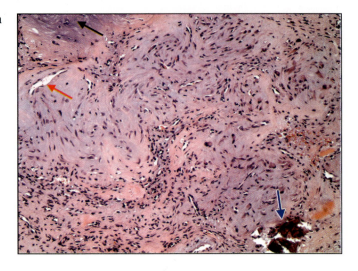

34. A 4-month-old boy presents with a 1.6 cm mass above the left knee. No evidence of muscle infiltration is seen. The radiologic differential diagnosis includes benign fibroma or old hematoma. What is the correct diagnosis?
    (a) Infantile fibrosarcoma
    (b) Myxoinflammatory fibroblastic sarcoma
    (c) Inflammatory myofibroblastic tumor
    (d) Solitary fibrous tumor
    (e) Infantile fibromatosis

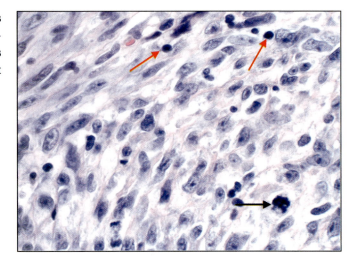

35. A 63-year-old man injured his right ring finger 2 years ago and now has a 0.4 cm nodule at the site. What is the correct diagnosis?
    (a) Neuroma
    (b) Morton's neuroma
    (c) Neurofibroma
    (d) Traumatic neuroma
    (e) Ganglioneuroma

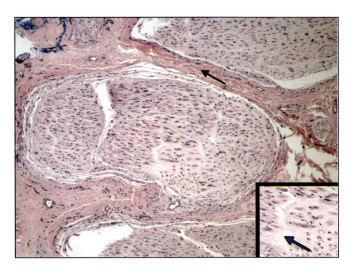

36. A newborn has multiple lesions with this histologic appearance. What site for the lesions has been shown to be associated with up to 75% mortality?
(a) Soft tissue of extremities
(b) Ribcage
(c) Lung and heart
(d) Brain
(e) Genitals

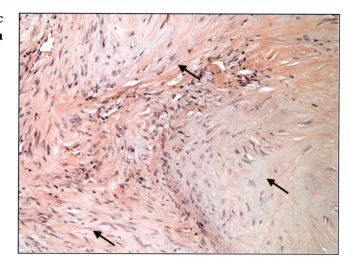

37. A 16-year-old male with a history of a left parates-ticular malignancy which was resected and treated with chemoradiation now has a retroperitoneal mass that stains positively for MyoD1. What is the correct diagnosis?
(a) MPNST (triton tumor)
(b) Embryonal rhabdomyosarcoma, classic type
(c) Embryonal rhabdomyosarcoma, spindle cell type
(d) Dedifferentiated liposarcoma
(e) Leiomyosarcoma

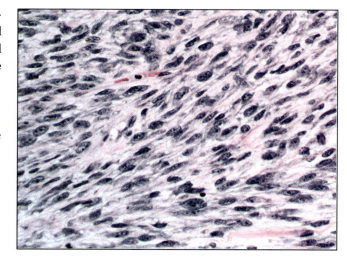

38. A 16-year-old boy has a 0.5 cm nodule on his left posterior thigh. What is the correct diagnosis?
(a) Dermatofibroma
(b) Myxoid neurothekeoma
(c) Cellular neurothekeoma
(d) Atypical fibroxanthoma
(e) Myxofibrosarcoma

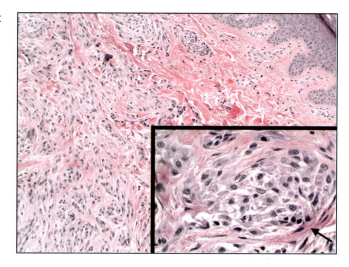

39. A 22-year-old man has a mid tibial medullary lesion with a groundglass appearance on X-ray. What is the correct diagnosis for this lesion depicted to the right?

(a) Ossifying fibroma

(b) Non-ossifying fibroma

(c) Monostotic fibrous dysplasia

(d) Osteofibrous dysplasia

(e) Parosteal osteosarcoma

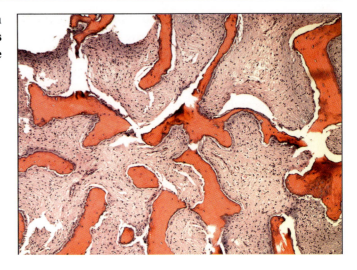

40. A 63-year-old wheelchair bound female has a 6 cm buttock lesion. What is the correct diagnosis?

(a) Decubitus ulcer

(b) Malignant melanoma

(c) Hodgkin's lymphoma

(d) Systemic amyloidosis

(e) Ischemic fasciitis

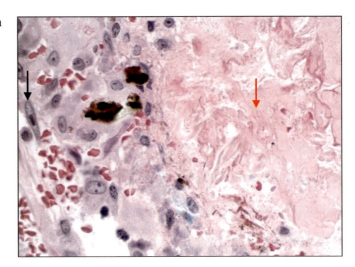

41. A 57-year-old female has a right arm 2 cm dermal nodule with histology as shown to the right. Tumor cells stain positively for EMA but negatively for S-100. What is the correct diagnosis?

(a) Dermatofibroma

(b) Leiomyoma

(c) Schwannoma

(d) Neurofibroma

(e) Perineurioma

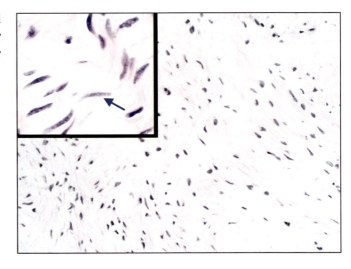

42. **At birth, a male neonate has a 1 cm tongue mass. What is the correct diagnosis?**
   (a) Embryonal rhabdomyosarcoma, classic variant
   (b) Fetal rhabdomyoma, intermediate type
   (c) Fetal rhabdomyoma, myxoid type
   (d) Adult rhabdomyoma
   (e) Fibrous hamartoma of infancy

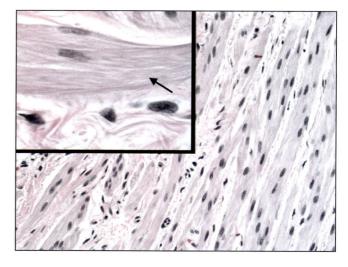

43. **A 39-year-old female has a growing soft tissue mass on the inner border of her second left toe. What is the correct diagnosis?**
   (a) Well-differentiated liposarcoma
   (b) Fibrolipoma
   (c) Spindle cell lipoma
   (d) Lipoma
   (e) Lipoblastoma

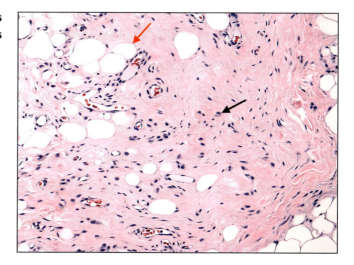

44. **An EVG stain is shown in the inset. What is the most common site of this lesion?**
   (a) Mouth
   (b) Shoulder
   (c) Periscapular
   (d) Retroperitoneal
   (e) Sole of foot

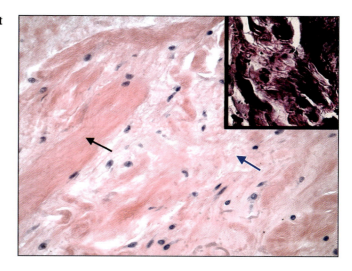

45. A 57-year-old female has a 1.4 cm extra-axial mass abutting the right superior cerebellar peduncle in the right tentorial incisura. The tumor cells stain positively for CD34 and CD99. What is the correct diagnosis?

  (a) Solitary fibrous tumor

  (b) Meningioma, fibroblastic variant

  (c) Ewing Sarcoma

  (d) Synovial sarcoma

  (e) Fibrosarcoma

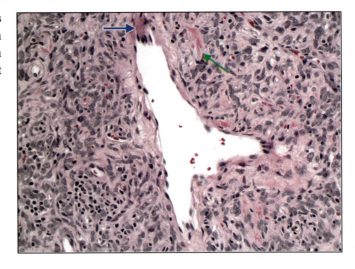

46. A 19-year-old male has an L3 intradural lesion. Histology from the lesion is shown to the right. What is the correct diagnosis?

  (a) Melanotic schwannoma

  (b) Metastatic melanoma

  (c) Melanotic neuroectodermal tumor of infancy

  (d) Metastatic papillary thyroid carcinoma

  (e) Nonossifying fibroma

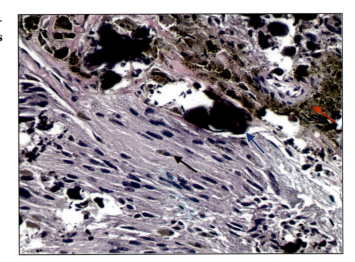

47. A 71-year-old man with a history of left ear melanoma has a 1 cm parotid lesion shown to the right. An FNA is nondiagnostic. What stain will highlight this lesion?

  (a) Melan-A

  (b) AE1/AE3

  (c) Alcian blue

  (d) CD34

  (e) Desmin

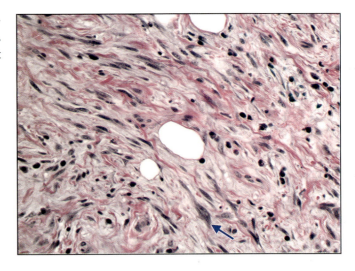

48. This lesion in an infant is associated with which of the following syndromes?
(a) Terminal osseous dysplasia
(b) Oral-facial-digital syndrome
(c) Incontinentia pigmenti
(d) Velocardialfacial syndrome
(e) Turner's syndrome

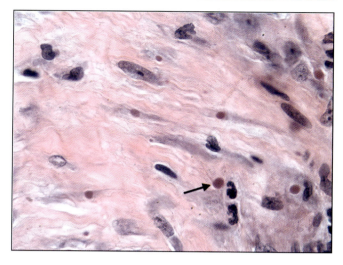

49. A 48-year-old man has a 7 cm left posterior chest wall lesion. What is the correct diagnosis?
(a) Low grade fibromyxoid sarcoma
(b) Myxofibrosarcoma
(c) Elastofibroma
(d) Fibromatosis involving muscle
(e) Desmoplastic fibroblastoma

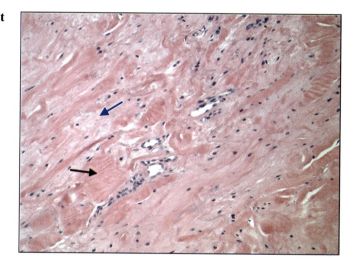

50. A 51-year-old patient has a right trigger thumb. A cystic lesion was found at trigger thumb release surgery. What is the correct diagnosis?
(a) Fibromatosis
(b) Dermatofibroma
(c) Ganglion cyst
(d) Myofibromatosis
(e) Fibroma of tendon sheath

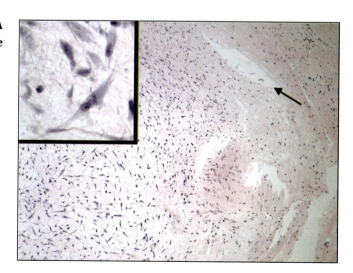

51. **A 47-year-old has a 6 cm retroperitoneal mass. What is the correct diagnosis?**
   (a) Spindle cell lipoma
   (b) Angiolipoma
   (c) Angiomyolipoma
   (d) Myolipoma
   (e) Myelolipoma

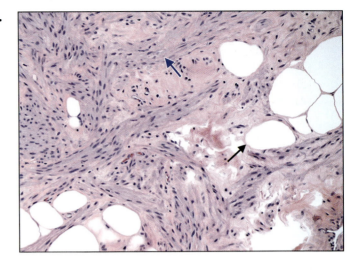

52. **A 40-year-old female has a 7 cm calcified left thigh mass that stains positively for desmin. What is the correct diagnosis?**
   (a) Synovial sarcoma
   (b) Leiomyoma of deep soft tissue
   (c) Symplastic leiomyoma
   (d) STUMP
   (e) Leiomyosarcoma

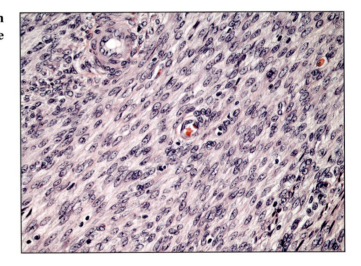

53. **A perirenal mass is found in a 52-year-old woman with the histology shown to the right. What clinical syndrome is this lesion most closely associated with?**
   (a) Cowden syndrome
   (b) Carney's triad
   (c) Neurofibromatosis 2
   (d) Sturge-Weber syndrome
   (e) Tuberous sclerosis

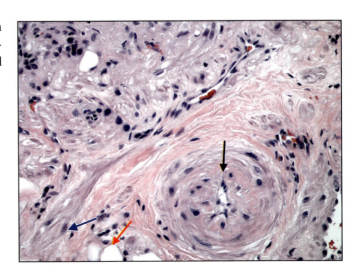

54. If this lesion were from a 2.7 cm lesion in the soft tissue of the second phalanx of a 26-year-old man, what would the correct diagnosis be?
  (a) Fibro-osseous pseudotumor of digits
  (b) Myositis ossificans
  (c) Chondroma
  (d) Osteosarcoma
  (e) Chondrosarcoma

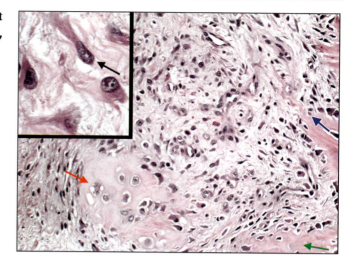

55. A 39-year-old male has a soft tissue mass in the right vastus lateral muscle. What is the correct diagnosis?
  (a) Elastofibroma
  (b) Myxoid chondrosarcoma
  (c) Desmoplastic fibroblastoma
  (d) Fibrosarcoma
  (e) Fibromatosis

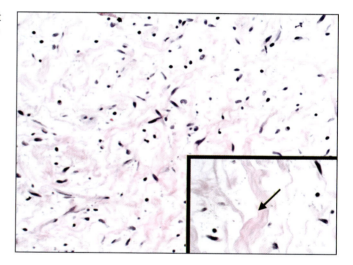

56. A 39-year-old man has a left elbow lesion. What is the correct diagnosis?
  (a) Leiomyoma
  (b) Myxoma
  (c) Myofibroma
  (d) Myofibroblastoma
  (e) Fibroma

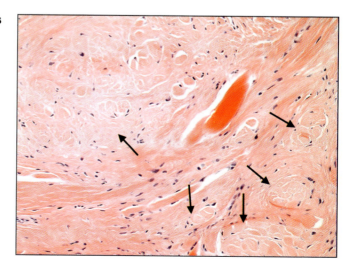

57. This lesion is found in the deep abdominal dermis of a 45-year-old man. What stain is it most likely to be positive for?

(a) Desmin

(b) CD99

(c) S-100

(d) CD34

(e) C-kit

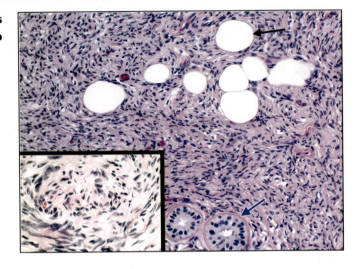

58. A 30-year-old man has a tibial midshaft lytic medullary lesion shown to the right. Which cytogenetic changes are likely to be present in the lesional cells?

(a) Trisomies in chromosomes 7, 8, 12, 19, and 21

(b) Ring chromosomes and giant marker chromosomes

(c) Multiple complex cytogenetic changes

(d) T(17;22)

(e) T(12;16)

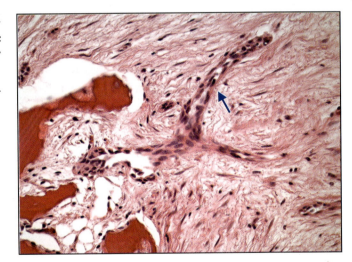

59. A 9-year-old has a mass of the right elbow. The cells are vimentin positive but S-100 negative. What is the correct diagnosis?

(a) Infantile fibrosarcoma

(b) Infantile fibromatosis

(c) MPNST

(d) Myofibromatosis

(e) Fetal rhabdomyoma

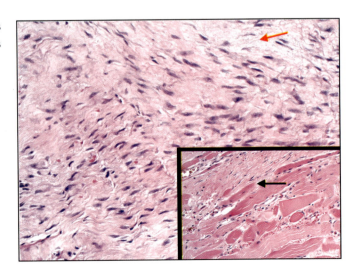

60. **This lesion, in a patient with a strong cancer family history, is seen infiltrating fat. What is the patient's prognosis?**
    (a) Over 40% lifetime risk of gastric cancer
    (b) Near 100% lifetime risk of colon cancer
    (c) Over 40% lifetime risk of breast cancer
    (d) Multiple cutaneous nevoid basal cell carcinomas
    (e) Increased risk of peripancreatic neuroendocrine neoplasms.

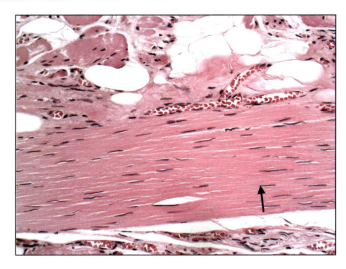

61. **An 8-year-old male has a 1 cm mass at the distal aspect of the third left phalanx. What is the correct diagnosis?**
    (a) Infantile digital fibroma
    (b) Inclusion body fibromatosis
    (c) Dupuytren's contracture
    (d) Desmoid fibromatosis
    (e) Fibrosarcoma

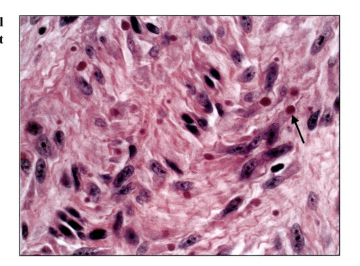

62. **A 41-year-old man has been followed for a decade for a left tibial mass. Radiologically it is a 16.8 cm lobulated enhancing mass wrapping around the medial aspect of the proximal tibia. Edema is noted and muscle is displaced. What is the correct diagnosis?**
    (a) Periosteal osteosarcoma
    (b) Parosteal osteosarcoma
    (c) Conventional osteosarcoma
    (d) Fibrous dysplasia
    (e) Nonossifying fibroma

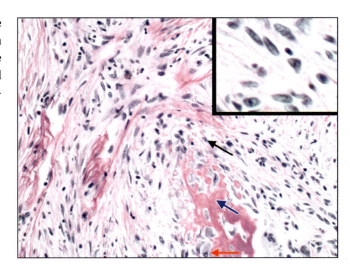

63. A 43-year-old man has a painless nodule on his right cheek depicted to the right. What stain most likely highlights the tumor cells?

(a) SMA

(b) Desmin

(c) HMB45

(d) S-100

(e) AE1/AE3

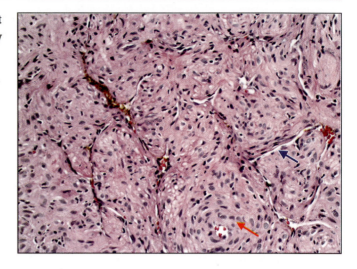

64. A 55-year-old man has a dermal nodule in the left groin. What is the correct diagnosis?

(a) Dermatofibroma

(b) DFSP

(c) Neurothekeoma

(d) Malignant melanoma

(e) Neurofibroma

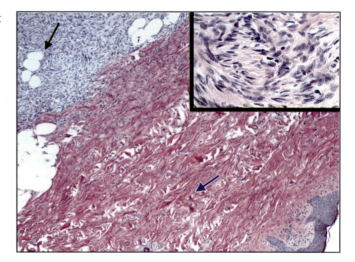

ANSWERS

1. **(c) EBV-associated smooth muscle tumor**
   This lesion occurs in individuals that have been immunosuppressed for any reason including due to HIV or steroid use. Histologically, fascicles of bland spindled myofibroblasts with eosinophilic cytoplasm are seen. The postiive EBER stain in the setting of a patient with HIV makes EBV-associated smooth muscle tumor the correct diagnosis. The other answer choices are not associated with EBER positivity.

2. **(c) Nodular Kaposi sarcoma**
   Nodular Kaposi sarcoma is characterized by nodules of spindled cells (black arrow) with cells containing clear cytoplasm or slit like vessels, creating a sieve-like pattern. The spindled cells are uniform without prominent cytologic atypia. Associated with the spindled nodules in Kaposi sarcoma is an exuberant chronic inflammatory infiltrate (yellow arrow). Many cases of nodular Kaposi sarcoma also contain hyaline globules (red arrow). Patch-stage Kaposi sarcoma features a proliferation of small vessels surrounding ectatic vessels with little spindling component. Nodular architecture like that seen here is more consistent with nodular Kaposi sarcoma. While benign inflammatory cells are seen, the nodule of spindled cells is not consistent with granulomatous inflammation which would not show clear cytoplasm and such an organized, fascicular arrangement of spindled cells. Kaposiform hemangioendothelioma would show a capillary component in addition to the spindled cells seen here.

3. **(e) Myofibroma**
   Myofibroma can be characterized by alternating light-appearing hypocellular regions and dark-appearing hypercellular regions (blue arrow). The hypocellular areas tend to have a vaguely nodular appearance (black arrow) which can lead to diagnostic confusion with granulomatous lesions. However, the cells are not histiocytic; instead, they are bland and spindled ruling out granulomatous inflammation. There is no necrosis and epithelioid sarcoma almost never occurs on the face. The absence of necrobiotic collagen rules out granuloma annulare. The alternating cellularity and nodularity is reminiscent of a degenerating leiomyoma; however, desmin negativity and the lack of a fascicular architecture rules against leiomyoma. SMA positivity and desmin negativity is typical of myofibroma.

4. **(b) Ancient schwannoma**
   Ancient schwannomas have a similar low power histologic appearance to normal schwannoma, featuring a fibrous capsule (black arrow) encapsulating hypocellular Antoni B areas (blue arrow) and hypercellular Antoni A areas (red arrow). The inset shows severe cytologic atypia present in the Antoni A areas. This is called ancient change and is a form of benign degeneration with a minimal chance of metastasis or recurrence. Fibromatosis is not encapsulated and would feature bland spindled cells without the cytologic atypia seen here. Neurofibroma, plexiform neurofibroma, and malignant peripheral nerve sheath tumor would not be encapsulated.

5. **(b) Beta-catenin**
   The lesion depicted is desmoid fibromatosis. Distinctive features include the investment of muscle fibers (black arrow) by a paucicellular population of bland fibrous cells (blue arrow). Beta catenin stains over 90% of desmoid fibromatoses. Desmin is rarely positive. AE1/AE3, CD34, and S-100 are consistently negative.

6. **(a) Infantile digital fibroma**
   This lesion depicts spindled fibroblasts some of which exhibit ganglion-like characteristics (red arrow), characteristic of but not specific for infantile digital fibroma. Scattered eosinophilic inclusions are seen (black arrow) that narrow the differential diagnosis to infantile digital fibroma versus inclusion body fibromatosis. The location of the lesion (digital) and the age of the patient (infant age range) make infantile digital fibroma the correct diagnosis.

7. **(c) Ganglioneuroma**
   A mixture of mature ganglion cells (blue arrow) and interweaving mildly spindled and wavy schwannian cells (red arrow) are seen, diagnostic of ganglioneuroma in the absence of an immature element. Ganglion cells are

distinctive due to their large size, voluminous cytoplasm, eccentric nuclei, and occasional prominent nucleoli. No small round blue cells are present which would be necessary for a diagnosis of neuroblastoma or ganglioneuroblastoma. Malignant melanoma would be more cellular and atypical. Plasma cell neoplasm is unlikely since the ganglion cells are far larger than the size of a plasma cell.

8. **(b) Inflammatory myofibroblastic tumor**

The clinical history of a well-circumscribed lesion with a history of fever raise suspicion for inflammatory myofibroblastic tumor (IMT). Histologically, a considerable lymphoid infiltrate (red arrow) along with spindled ganglion-like myofibroblasts (black arrow) in a fascicular arrangement support the diagnosis of IMT. ALK positivity is seen in approximately half of these tumors. There is not enough nuclear pleomorphism for a diagnosis of inflammatory pleomorphic undifferentiated sarcoma or myxoinflammatory fibroblastic sarcoma. The histopathology of this lesion is not in keeping with Hodgkin's lymphoma or anaplastic large cell lymphoma which also stains positively for ALK.

9. **(a) Nodular fasciitis**

This image depicts the tissue culture-type appearance of nodular fasciitis. Immature spindled fibroblasts are seen with oval shaped nuclei and distal tapering. Ischemic fasciitis would display large areas of necrosis. Fibromatosis would display a less haphazard, more fasciular arrangement of spindled cells without distal tapering. Low grade fibromyxoid sarcoma would have some clearly myxoid areas adjoining fibrous areas. Myofibromatosis would feature nodules of myofibroblasts which are not seen.

10. **(c) Desmoid fibromatosis**

The image depicts mature adipose tissue being infiltrated by an aggressive spindle cell lesion (black arrow). The spindled cells are bland, monotonous, and the nuclei are relatively well spaced from each other, making fibrosarcoma unlikely and supporting the diagnosis of desmoid fibromatosis. Myofibroma would show a more nodular appearance. In fibrolipoma, the fibrous tissue has haphazardly distributed nuclei, not the fascicular arrangement shown in the picture. Schwannoma would show Antoni A and B zones and would be encapsulated.

11. **(d) Low grade myofibroblastic sarcoma**

This image shows a low grade myofibroblastic sarcoma. These lesions are composed of eosinophilic spindled cells with mild nuclear atypia. As seen in this case, they most commonly affect the head and neck regions of middle aged adults. Focal invasion of lamellar bone is present (blue arrow), highlighting the malignant nature of this lesion. There is not enough cellularity for a fibrosarcoma and the immunoprofile does not fit. Osteosarcoma would feature immature osteoid formation; however, the bone we see in the image is mature lamellar bone, indicating that the bone is a bystander and not part of the malignant process. Fibrous dysplasia is unlikely with the bony infiltration seen, mild atypia, and staining pattern. Leiomyosarcoma is a close differential. Histologically, both tumors have cigar-shaped spindled eosinophilic cells and both can stain positively for smooth muscle actin and desmin. However, only low grade myofibroblastic sarcoma stains negative for h-caldesmon.

12. **(c) Desmoplastic fibroma**

Desmoplastic fibroma of bone is an expansile destructive lesion often found in the metaphyses of long bones or the mandible. The target demographic is young adults in their second to third decades. Desmoplastic fibroma is the bone version of soft tissue fibromatosis since the two are microscopically identical, showing bland fibroblasts distributed in a densely collagenous stroma. Since this is a bone lesion not a soft tissue lesion, fibromatosis is not correct. Nonossifying fibroma would have foam cells, giant cells, and hemosiderin laden macrophages. Low grade fibrosarcoma would show a herringbone pattern with slight atypia which is not seen here. Well-differentiated intramedullary osteosarcoma would also show at least minimal atypia and tumor bone formation.

13. **(a) Schwannoma**

This is an encapsulated (red arrow) lesion composed of sparsely populated spindle cells. The spindled cells show mild atypia also known as early ancient change (blue arrow); scattered inflammatory cells are seen (black arrow). These findings are characteristic of schwannoma which in this case is almost entirely composed of hypocellular Antoni B areas. In other schwannomas, Antoni A areas with verocay bodies can be seen. Some of the other choices can be close histologic mimics but none would display such a prominent capsule.

14. (b) CD34

This is a spindle cell lipoma characterized by a proliferation of bland spindled cells (black arrow) in a background of adipocytes (red arrow). CD34 strongly and diffusely stains the spindled cells of spindle cell lipoma. S-100 would stain the adipocytes but would be negative in the spindled cells. Factor XIIIA is a marker for fibroblasts which highlights cells in dermatofibroma. However, dermatofibroma is known for collagen entrapment and a more superficial location. Spindle cell lipoma shows only focal staining for Factor XIIIA. Actin and desmin are negative in spindle cell lipoma.

15. (b) Myofibroblastoma

Myofibroblastoma of the breast features fascicles of bland spindled cells (red arrow) which are separated by thick collagen ribbons (black arrow). Dermatofibroma is a similar lesion that contains collagen trapping, a feature that the collagen ribbons can mimic. However, CD34 is positive in this and most myofibroblastomas, inconsistent with a dermatofibroma. Dermatofibrosarcoma protuberans (DFSP) is positive for CD34 but would show fat and adnexal entrapment instead with a storiform architecture that is not seen here. Spindle cell lipoma shares the loss of 13q14 with myofibroblastoma of breast and has a similar spindled cell population. However, no significant adipocytic population is seen in the image. Angiomyofibroblastoma would feature spindled or epithelioid cells radiating out from vessels which is not seen here.

16. (c) Juvenile hyaline fibromatosis

This image depicts juvenile hyaline fibromatosis in which randomly distributed bland cells are embedded in an eosinophilic matrix (black arrow). Patients with this lesion often have a clinical syndrome of joint contractures, gingival hyperplasia, and multiple skin lesions featuring the eosinophilic matrix seen in the image. Neurothekeoma and myxoid chondrosarcoma feature a more nodular, septated growth pattern. Myxofibrosarcoma would display cytologic atypia. A myxoma would have stroma that is more edematous and less eosinophilic.

17. (c) Calcifying aponeurotic fibroma

Calcifying aponeurotic fibroma depicts foci of calcifications (red arrow), bland fibroblasts, and occasional cells with a cartilaginous appearance (blue arrow) embedded in a dense collagenous stroma (black arrow). Fibromatosis is unlikely to have calcifications or a chondroid appearance. Chondroma is more well-circumscribed and should not have the fibroblastic cells seen here. Calciphylaxis is seen in the setting of renal failure and would feature vascular calcium deposition not seen here. Chondrosarcoma with dystrophic calcifications would have a cartilaginous matrix, not individual chondrocytes deposited in a fibrous matrix.

18. (e) Cellular schwannoma

The lesion shows a thick fibrous capsule (black arrow) entrapping a nodule of spindled cells (blue arrow) consistent with Antoni A regions in a cellular schwannoma. Along with the capsule and spindled cells, S-100 positivity also supports the diagnosis of cellular schwannoma. GIST will stain negatively for S-100. Wilm's tumor would show a small round blue cell component occasionally mixed with epithelial cells which are not seen. Neuroblastoma is a small round blue cell tumor and should not show spindling. Neurofibroma is not encapsulated.

19. (a) Dermatofibroma

Dermatofibroma shows a dermal spindle cell population composed of fibroblasts and epithelioid histiocytes that features collagen entrapment (black arrow). Spindled cells are bland with minimal cytologic atypia. Subcutical involvement is rarely present as this is a benign tumor. DFSP would show a storiform appearance and honeycomb-wrapping around fat. Neurothekeoma would show fibrous septae between nodules. Neurofibroma would show wavy spindled cells suggestive of neural differentiation. Scar would show parallel fascicles of bland spindled cells.

20. (c) Desmin

This is a myolipoma. The image shows the characteristic interweaving fascicles of eosinophilic cells (blue arrow) associated with mature adipose tissue (black arrow) that is typical for this lesion. The retroperitoneum is a common site for myolipoma which can grow to be even larger than the 9 cm one described in this case. The smooth muscle fascicles stain positively for the smooth muscle markers desmin and smooth muscle actin. CD34 highlights the spindled cells in DFSP and spindle cell lipoma. However, the retroperitoneum is an uncommon site for DFSP and spindle cell lipoma cells would not be so fascicular. CD99 highlights monophasic synovial sarcoma which would have more pleomorphism and cellularity. S-100 would label a neurofibroma which would not feature mature adipocytes.

21. **(b) NF1**

A proliferation of large dilated nerve fibers are seen in the image with diffuse myxoid changes (black arrow), diagnostic of plexiform neurofibroma. Most plexiform neurofibroma patients have NF1, a syndrome caused by a mutation in neurofibromin 1. This syndrome is characterized by café au lait spots, Lisch nodules in the eye, musculoskeletal pathology, mental retardation, and increased benign skin tumors like that seen in this case, among other clinical abnormalities. Some plexiform neurofibromas can undergo malignant transformation into malignant peripheral nerve sheath tumor, a significant cause of death in NF1 patients. The other answer choices are not associated with plexiform neurofibromas.

22. **(c) Carney complex**

This melanotic schwannoma has a typical presentation, arising in the midline of a young adult. The histologic features of spindled cells (blue arrow), psammomatous calcifications (red arrow), and pigment deposition (green arrow) are all present. Melanotic schwannoma is associated with Carney syndrome, which includes melanotic schwannoma, myxomas, dermal lentigines and nevi, and endocrine overactivity. The other answer choices are not associated with melanotic schwannoma.

23. **(c) Nuclear beta-catenin**

The lesion shown is an infantile digital fibroma. Characteristic histologic findings include adnexal entrapment by bland fibroblasts (black arrow) and a fibroblastic dermal proliferation that appears to extend all the way to the dermal-epidermal junction. A specific feature found in the question stem is the presence of eosinophilic inclusions at high power. Nuclear beta-catenin is negative in cases of infantile digital fibroma but positive in cases of adult fibromatosis. The other stains are positive in most infantile digital fibroma cases.

24. **(b) Traumatic neuroma**

Traumatic neuroma contains haphazardly irregularly oriented small nerve fascicles (blue arrow) in a fibrous background (black arrow). These lesions occur after trauma or surgery as in this case. Neurofibroma, leiomyoma, and schwannoma would not feature fascicles of nerves in a fibrous stroma. Mucosal neuroma would feature larger nerve bundles surrounded by a perineurium and a myxoid background, which is not seen here.

25. **(b) Neurofibroma**

An unencapsulated dermal population of small spindled cells are seen some of which display wavy nuclei (black arrow), suggestive of neural differentation; with S-100 positivity this is a neurofibroma. Dermatofibroma and DFSP would not stain for S-100. A schwannoma would show a capsule. Perineurioma would stain negatively for S-100.

26. **(b) Myofibromatosis**

Myofibromatosis typically occurs in children under the age of two. The image shows multiple sparsely cellular nodules (black arrows) of bland myofibroblasts with eosinophilic cytoplasm. These findings are consistent with myofibroma. However, the presence of multiple nodules merits the diagnosis of myofibromatosis. Congenital fibrosarcoma would not be nodular and would show more cellularity with scattered inflammatory cells. Hemangiopericytoma would show staghorn vessels and would be less nodular. Fibrous hamartoma of infancy would show mature adipose tissue intermixed with intersecting myofibroblastic fascicles and alcian blue positive regions, none of which is seen.

27. **(c) CD34**

This lesion is dermatofibroma. Note the collagen entrapment by a bland population of spindle cells (black arrow). The malignant counterpart to a dermatofibroma is dermatofibrosarcoma protuberans. CD34 is the only stain listed that stains negatively in dermatofibroma but positively in dermatofibrosarcoma protuberans. Both tumors stain negatively for S-100, desmin, and pancytokeratin. They both stain positively for vimentin.

28. **(d) Proliferative myositis**

Proliferative myositis most commonly affects the central and peripheral upper body with the shoulder being a common preferred site. A large fraction of cases include a history of some trauma as in the question stem. Histologically, myofibroblasts (red arrow) infiltrating skeletal muscle (black arrow) are seen. A key component is the presence of ganglion-like cells with abundant light amphophilic cytoplasm and eccentric nuclei (blue arrow). Ganglioneuroma would not typically involve skeletal muscle intimately as seen in this lesion. Ganglioneuroblastoma would have a small round blue immature component. Metastastic signet ring cell carcinoma would not feature a myofibroblastic proliferation. Nodular fasciitis would not have ganglion-like cells.

29. **(c) Fibrous hamartoma of infancy**

Fibrous hamartoma of infancy is characterized by cross-weaving fascicles of myofibroblasts (red arrow), benign mature adipocytes (green arrow), and alcian blue positive regions containing smaller cells (blue arrow). Gardner fibroma and nuchal type fibroma do not have fascicular myofibroblasts or alcian blue regions. Myofibroma has a more nodular appearance to its myofibroblasts with no alcian blue positivity. Granuloma annulare has alcian blue positivity but is composed of alcian blue areas surrounded by palisading histiocytes, which are not seen here.

30. **(b) Dupuytren's contracture**

Dupuytren's contracture features nodules of bland spindled fibroblasts (black arrow) present in the hands. While, histologically, this is fibromatosis, consideration of the special site of the fibromatosis, the hands, yields the more specific diagnosis. Although myofibromatosis can exhibit a nodular architecture, adult myofibromatosis occurs in the head area or below the waist. The hand would be an unusual site. Low grade fibromyxoid sarcoma can feature similar nodules but the nodules are more edematous or myxoid in low grade fibromyxoid sarcoma. Low grade myofibroblastic sarcoma would demonstrate more atypia and would not be nodular.

31. **(d) Angiomyofibroblastoma**

Angiomyofibroblastoma is characterized by a dermal proliferation of sometimes dilated vessels (black arrow) in a matrix of epithelioid or spindled cells (blue arrow) radiating out from vessels. This is the correct site for a cellular angiofibroma; however, cellular angiofibroma often is more fascicular and would not show the spindled cells radiating out from vessels as seen here. Angiomyxoma also could occur in this location; however, the stroma would be more edematous and paucicellular than that seen in this image, without radiating fibroblasts. Dermatofibroma features collagen trapping, not spindled cells surrounding vessels which is seen here. Lobular capillary hemangioma does not have a prominent spindle cell component.

32. **(a) Loss of 16q, 13q**

This is a spindle cell lipoma. The image depicts the typical histologic findings of adipocytes (red arrow) with a varied amount of spindled, bland cells (blue arrow) interspersed. Spindle cell lipomas are characterized by deletions on the long arms of chromosomes 13 and 16 (13q and 16q). Ring chromosomes and giant marker chromosomes are atypical chromosomes associated with well-differentiated liposarcoma. This is not a well-differentiated liposarcoma because of the lack of nuclear irregularities and the lack of lipoblasts. Pleomorphic liposarcoma is typified by complex multifocal cytogenetic changes and the nuclei here are too bland for that to be the correct diagnosis.

33. **(a) Vimentin**

This is a phosphaturic mesenchymal tumor. Diagnostic features include the chondromyxoid matrix with a basophilic hue (black arrow), numerous irregularly shaped vessels (red arrow), and calcifications (blue arrow). Vimentin is the only stain listed that reliably highlights phosphaturic mesenchymal tumor.

34. **(a) Infantile fibrosarcoma**

The image shows a cellular spindle cell proliferation in a herringbone pattern, that is found in both infantile fibrosarcoma and adult fibrosarcoma. Tumor infiltrating lymphocytes (red arrow) and a high mitotic rate (black arrow) are features that support the diagnosis of infantile fibrosarcoma. Myxoinflammatory fibroblastic sarcoma would feature more cytologic atypia with bizarre cells. In inflammatory myofibroblastic tumor, the lymphocytes would be more concentrated and a herringbone pattern would not be typical for IMT. Neither solitary fibrous tumor nor infantile fibromatosis would have this amount of scattered lymphocytes.

35. **(a) Neuroma**

The histology demonstrated here is that of a neuroma with thick fibrous septae (black arrow) and large caliber nerve degeneration (blue arrow). Morton's neuroma is a term that applies to foot lesions, not finger lesions. Traumatic neuroma would feature a proliferation of nerve fascicles that is not seen here. The myxoid changes are focal and degenerative not diffuse as would be seen in plexiform neurofibroma. No ganglion cells are present, ruling out ganglioneuroma; additionally, ganglioneuroma most often affects axial sites such as the mediastinum or retroperitoneum.

36. **(c) Lung and heart**

Myofibromatosis in the lung, heart, and other visceral organs of a newborn has been associated with a high mortality rate. The depicted lesion is a myofibroma because there are three nodules of plump myofibroblasts (black arrows) with eosinophilic cytoplasm and a sparse distribution. The myofibroblasts display minimal cytologic atypia. The presence of multiple lesions makes this myofibromatosis.

37. **(c) Embryonal rhabdomyosarcoma, spindle cell type**

This lesion is an embryonal rhabdomyosarcoma, spindle cell type; however, without the myoD1 positivity, this diagnosis could not have been made. The image features eosinophilic spindled cells in a fascicular arrangement which is a nonspecific finding in the absence of MyoD1 positivity. Embryonal rhabdomyosarcoma, classic type, would have small round blue cells with an alternating hypocellular-hypercellular arrangement. Dedifferentiated liposarcoma can show rhabdomyoblastic differentiation but would be associated with a well-differentiated liposarcomatous component which is not seen. MPNST with rhabdomyoblastic differentiation (malignant triton tumor) would show rhabdomyoblasts with eccentric nuclei and abundant eosinophilic cytoplasm instead of the spindled cells seen here. The MyoD1 positivity and lack of severe atypia rule out leiomyosarcoma.

38. **(c) Cellular neurothekeoma**

Cellular neurothekeoma shows a dermal proliferation of nodules composed of neoplastic epithelioid cells with amphophilic cytoplasm. Frequently nodules will be lined by fibrous septae (black arrow). These lesions tend to affect teenagers and are more common in the upper body than the lower body. With an ill-defined dermal lesion of cells with amphophilic cytoplasm, dermatofibroma comes into the differential diagnosis; however, dermatofibroma would not show the well-circumscribed lobules seen in this case. Many cellular neurothekeoma cases have a myxoid component; however, none is seen in this image, ruling out myxoid neurothekeoma and myxofibrosarcoma. There is insufficient atypia for atypical fibroxanthoma which also would not be nodular.

39. **(c) Monostotic fibrous dysplasia**

Fibrous dysplasia features a curvilinear distribution of bony trabeculae lining a population of bland spindled cells as seen in the image. The other answer choices comprise several histologic mimics of fibrous dysplasia that can be eliminated based on the presence or absence of osteoblastic rimming and the site of the lesion. The magnification is too low to discern osteoblastic rimming so location is the main tool that has to be used to get to the correct answer. Ossifying fibroma occurs most commonly in the jaw, not the tibia. Non-ossifying fibroma is a metaphyseal lesion, not a midshaft medullary lesion. Osteofibrous dysplasia does occur in the tibia but is a cortical not a medullary lesion. Parosteal osteosarcoma is located in the metaphysis or metaphysis-diaphysis juncture, not midshaft. This fibrous dysplasia is monostotic because it only involves one site.

40. **(e) Ischemic fasciitis**

More common in the pressurized soft tissues of wheelchair bound patients, the hallmarks of ischemic fasciitis are fibrinoid necrosis (red arrow) surrounded by ganglion-like fibroblasts (black arrow). The prominent nucleoli and hemosiderin deposition make malignant melanoma a diagnostic consideration; however, the nuclear regularity and the nature and extracellular location of the pigment (hemosiderin) make melanoma unlikely. There is no lymphocytic milieu that would be expected with Hodgkin's lymphoma. A sacral decubitus ulcer would show abundant acute inflammation that is not seen here. Systemic amyloidosis would display hyaline amyloid not fibrinoid necrosis and would not have a fibroblastic ganglion-like rim.

41. **(e) Perineurioma**

This perineurioma features a hypocellular proliferation of mildly fascicular spindled cells some of which display wavy nuclei (blue arrow) suggestive of neural differentiation. These findings are nonspecific and can be seen in neurofibroma as well. However, EMA positivity with S-100 negativity is not seen in any of the other answer choices.

42. (b) Fetal rhabdomyoma, intermediate type

The tongue is a frequent site of involvement by fetal rhabdomyoma, intermediate type. The lesion is characterized by interweaving fibers of benign appearing muscle with striations (black arrow), pink cytoplasm, and little to no myxoid stroma between fascicles. Embryonal rhabdomyosarcoma, classic variant, would not feature abundant eosinophilic cytoplasm as it is a small round blue cell tumor. Fetal rhabdomyoma, myxoid type, more common in this age group, would show more of a myxoid matrix between muscle fibers. Adult rhabdomyoma would have polygonal cells with abundant deep pink to red cytoplasm. Fibrous hamartoma of infancy would show interweaving myofibroblastic fascicles; however, it would also show mature fat and myxoid areas that are not seen here.

43. (c) Spindle cell lipoma

This image depicts the main features of spindle cell lipoma, adipocytes (red arrow) intermixed with various amounts of bland spindled cells which can be either haphazardly arranged (black arrow) or in parallel fascicles. The spindled cells are bland and there are no lipoblasts, making well-differentiated liposarcoma unlikely. Fibrolipoma would contain bland fibrous septae between adipocytes, not cellular haphazardly arranged spindled cells as seen here. A regular lipoma would exhibit mainly adipocytes with minimal interspersed fibrous tissue and no spindled population. An immature lipoblastoma could demonstrate spindled mesenchymal cells but would also show fibrous septae dividing adipocyte lobules that is not seen here.

44. (c) Periscapular

This lesion is an elastofibroma. It is typified by dense collagen fibrils (black arrow) interspersed by a collagenized hypocellular matrix (blue arrow). By far the most common location for elastofibroma is the periscapular region although elastofibromas in other areas have been reported.

45. (a) Solitary fibrous tumor

The picture depicts a staghorn (irregularly shaped) vessel with a hyalinized wall (blue arrow) surrounded by an architecture-less cellular proliferation of spindled cells, consistent with solitary fibrous tumor. Occasional collagen can be seen entrapped in the spindled cells of solitary fibrous tumor (green arrow). Fibroblastic meningioma would not show staghorn vessels. Ewing's sarcoma, fibrosarcoma, and synovial sarcoma would be negative for CD34.

46. (a) Melanotic schwannoma

This melanotic schwannoma displays a typical midline location and shows the usual histologic findings of fascicles of spindled cells (black arrow), psammomatous calcifications (blue arrow), and extensive pigment deposition (red arrow). Melanotic melanoma would not show psammomatous calcifications and would show more nuclear atypia. Melanotic neuroectodermal tumor of infancy is restricted to infants. Metastatic papillary thyroid carcinoma would show psammoma bodies but would have a more glandular architecture without pigment deposition. Nonossifying fibroma is a bone lesion and would show spindled cells and hemosiderin laden macrophages but would also show foam cells and would not have psammoma bodies.

47. (c) Alcian blue

This lesion shows streaming, tapering (blue arrow) spindled cells deposited in a myxoid background, all features of nodular fasciitis. Alcian blue is known to highlight the myxoid pools in nodular fasciitis. There is insufficient pleomorphism for melanoma or squamous cell carcinoma which would be marked by Melan-A and AE1/AE3 respectively. No hemangiopericytoma type vessels are seen to support a CD34-staining hemangiopericytoma. A desmin-staining leiomyoma would not have this myxoid background.

48. (a) Terminal osseous dysplasia

Terminal osseous dysplasia is a an X-linked syndrome which features skeletal dysplasia, abnormalities in pigmentation, and multiple digital fibromas similar to the one depicted here. It is associated with mutations in the FLNA gene. The image shows a bland proliferation of fibroblastic cells admixed with eosinophilic globular inclusions (black arrow). These inclusions are highly suggestive of infantile digital fibroma. The other syndromes are not associated with infantile digital fibroma.

49. (c) Elastofibroma

The image depicts the main features of elastofibroma: Thick fragmented elastic fibers (black arrow) embedded in a hypocellular collagenous stroma (blue arrow). These lesions most commonly occur in the periscapular region. Low grade fibromyxoid sarcoma and fibromatosis would have more cellularity and fascicular architecture to the spindled cells. Myxofibrosarcoma would show more pleomorphism. Desmoplastic fibroblastoma would not show thick fragmented elastic fibers.

50. (e) Fibroma of tendon sheath

As seen in the image, fibroma of tendon sheath features a well-circumscribed nodule of haphazardly sparsely distributed fibroblasts with spindled shapes in a fibrous or myxoid background. This tumor has a predilection for the hand joints in adults. These nodules often feature peripheral clefting (black arrow). Fibromatosis and myofibromatosis would not feature the peripheral clefting seen. Myofibromatosis would show pink myoid nodules not haphazard fibroblasts. Fibromatosis and dermatofibroma would be less circumscribed. Ganglion cyst does occur at joints but a thick fibrous capsule would be seen which is not present and a spindled population is not typical of ganglion cyst.

51. (d) Myolipoma

Myolipoma is composed of mature adipose tissue (black arrow) cross-hatched by interweaving fascicles of smooth muscle with eosinophilic cytoplasm (blue arrow). Angiolipoma would have vessels containing fibrin thrombi. Spindle cell lipoma would not contain smooth muscle. Angiomyolipoma would contain thick walled vessels. Myelolipoma would have bone marrow elements intermixed with mature adipose tissue

52. (b) Leiomyoma of deep soft tissue

This is a leiomyoma with fascicles of bland streaming cells and immunohistochemical evidence of smooth muscle differentiation (positive desmin stain). No atypia, necrosis, or discernible mitoses are present which could signify malignant potential. The deep extremity site makes this a leiomyoma of deep soft tissue which tends to occur in young to middle age adults in the deep extremities and is often calcified. Symplastic leiomyoma refers to uterine tumors with atypia but no mitoses or necrosis. There is no atypia present in this lesion which would occur in the other answer choices.

53. (e) Tuberous sclerosis

This image depicts thick walled vessels (black arrow), myoid perivascular cells (blue arrow), and mature adipocytes (red arrow). This triad is diagnostic of angiomyolipoma which is associated with tuberous sclerosis. The tumor cells can be highlighted by melanocytic and smooth muscle markers.

54. (a) Fibro-osseous pseudotumor of digits

This lesion has several features that can be found in reactive osteochondromatous proliferations such as Nora's lesion and fibro-osseous pseudotumor of digits, including osteoblastic rimming (blue arrow), woven bone (green arrow), spindled myofibroblasts (black arrow), and cartilaginous differentiation (red arrow). Given the site of the lesion and the histologic findings, fibro-osseous pseudotumor of digits is the correct diagnosis. Histologic findings are similar to that of myositis ossificans but no zoning is seen and myositis ossificans arises more commonly in muscle than in superficial soft tissues. The presence of woven bone is not consistent with chondroma and chondrosarcoma. The lack of atypia and hypocellularity of the specimen make osteosarcoma unlikely.

55. (c) Desmoplastic fibroblastoma

In desmoplastic fibroblastoma, bland spindled to stellate fibroblasts in a fibrous stroma form a vague matrix with cells and paucicellular "holes" between cells (black arrow). Fibrosarcoma and fibromatosis are more cellular, lacking the characteristic "holes". The site is not correct for elastofibroma, the collagen is not dense enough, and abundant elastic fibers are absent . Myxoid chondrosarcoma, while hypocellular, would show fibrous bands and cells with eosinophilic cytoplasm.

56. (c) Myofibroma

This lesion contains numerous small to large sized nodules (black arrows) populated by bland sparsely distributed myofibroblasts. The myofibroblasts have copious eosinophilic cytoplasm and spindled regular small nuclei. Myxoma would have a more edematous stroma. Leiomyoma would be more cellular and have a fascicular architecture. Myofibroblastoma contains fascicles of spindled cells separated by collagenous ribbons. The cellularity nearly replicates that of a fibroma; however, fibroma would not have the multinodular architecture seen here.

57. (d) CD34

DFSP (dermatofibrosarcoma protuberans) is found just below or in the dermis which is indicated by the presence of adnexal structures (blue arrow). DFSP is known to entrap but not destroy adipocytes (black arrow) and adnexal structures (blue arrow). The adipocytes are entrapped in a honeycomb manner. Additionally, the inset shows a storiform pattern that is consistent with DFSP. DFSP is known to stain positively for CD34 in over 90% of cases. Desmin would highlight a leiomyosarcoma; however, coagulative necrosis and atypia are not present. S-100 would stain a schwannoma but this lesion is not encapsulated. C-kit would highlight a metastatic GIST which would not characteristically show fat/adnexal trapping.

58. (a) Trisomies in chromosomes 7, 8, 12, 19, and 21

Adamantinomas occur in younger patients with an average age around 30. The most common site by far is the tibia, midshaft, where greater than 50% of adamantinomas are found. Histologically, irregularly shaped bland epithelial nests (blue arrow) are deposited in a bland spindled fibrous stroma with nearby bony trabeculae. Cytogenetically, these tumors are typified by trisomies that have been reported in chromosomes 7, 8, 12, 19, and 21. Ring chromosomes and giant marker chromosomes are found in well-differentiated liposarcoma which would show mature adipocytes with occasional atypical nuclei. Multiple complex cytogenetic changes are seen in high grade sarcomas like undifferentiated pleomorphic sarcoma; however, there is insufficient atypia here for that diagnosis. T(17;22) is found in DFSP and t(12;16) is seen in myxoid liposarcoma, neither of which would have epithelial nests.

59. (b) Infantile fibromatosis

Infantile fibromatosis is characterized by a bland, vaguely fascicular spindle cell proliferation that has focal myxoid areas (red arrow) and demonstrates locally invasive behavior, infiltrating and investing muscle (black arrow). This is the so-called desmoid type of infantile fibromatosis which typically occurs in children over the age of 5. Infantile fibrosarcoma is unlikely due to the lack of lymphocytic infiltrate and relatively low cellularity. Myofibromatosis features a more nodular appearance to the spindled myofibroblasts. Fetal rhabdomyoma shows striated spindled cells suggestive of smooth muscle differentiation which are not seen here. S-100 negativity and the lack of cytologic atypia makes MPNST unlikely.

60. (b) Near 100% lifetime risk of colon cancer

The lesion depicted is desmoid fibromatosis. Note the fascicular arrangement of regularly spaced, bland spindled cells (black arrow) infiltrating into fat. Desmoid fibromatosis is associated with mutations in the *APC* gene which causes familial adenomatous polyposis (FAP) syndrome. The patient's strong cancer family history lends additional evidence that this patient suffers from FAP which features autosomal dominant inheritance. FAP uniformly leads to the development of colorectal carcinomas. Choice A refers to mutations in the *CDH1* gene. Choice C refers to mutations in the *BRCA* gene. Choice D refers to Nevoid basal cell carcinoma syndrome or Gorlin syndrome. Choice E refers to the MEN 1 syndrome.

61. (b) Inclusion body fibromatosis

This lesion depicts a fascicular growth pattern common to fibromatosis and even fibrosarcoma. The clues to the correct diagnosis are in the question stem and in the presence of the eosinophilic inclusions (black arrow). Fibrosarcoma, desmoid fibromatosis, and Dupuytren's contracture do not have the eosinophilic inclusions. Infantile digital fibroma and inclusion body fibromatosis are histologically equivalent; however, infantile digital fibroma occurs in infants and on the digits. This patient's age supports the diagnosis of inclusion body fibromatosis.

62. (b) Parosteal osteosarcoma

Based on the radiologic findings, there should be high suspicion for parosteal osteosarcoma. Parosteal osteosarcoma has a predilection to encircle bone in the distal femur or proximal tibia as in this case. Histologically, foci of woven bone are seen (blue arrow) with osteoblastic rimming (red arrow) entrapped and infiltrated by long fascicles of bland spindled cells with low levels of cytologic atypia (black arrow). Periosteal osteosarcoma would have more of a cartilaginous component. Conventional osteosarcoma would show more cytologic atypia. Fibrous dysplasia is a medullary lesion and would not show osteoblastic rimming. Nonossifying fibroma would not show immature bone formation.

63. **(a) SMA**

    This is a myopericytoma with nodules of pink slightly spindled cells (red arrow) surrounding irregularly shaped vessels (blue arrow). Myopericytomas stain positively for smooth muscle actin in nearly all cases. 15% of cases stain positively for desmin and no staining has been reported for HMB45, S-100, and AE1/AE3.

64. **(b) DFSP**

    DFSP, or dermtofibrosarcoma protuberans, as shown in the picture, features an uninvolved dermal grenz-zone between the lesion and the epidermis (blue arrow) as well as a deep dermal hypercellular lesion composed of closely packed spindled cells which invest fat in a so-called honeycombed fashion (black arrow). The inset shows a high power view demonstrating the occasionally storiform architecture of the cytologically bland spindled cells that make up the lesion. Dermatofibroma is not as cellular and does not entrap fat; instead, it entraps collagen which is not seen here. Neurothekeoma occurs in the skin as well and would feature tumor nodules with fibrous septae separating lobules which are not seen here. Malignant melanoma is not characterized by a grens zone and would demonstrate melanin granules, increased cellularity, and nuclear pleomorphism. Neurofibroma is typically not as cellular as the lesion shown in the figure and is not known for storiform architecture.

CHAPTER 2

Pleomorphic Lesions

1. **A 60-year-old female has a left infrascapular cyst. What is the correct diagnosis?**
   - (a) Giant cell tumor of soft parts
   - (b) Elastofibroma
   - (c) Giant cell fibroblastoma
   - (d) Chemotherapy atypia
   - (e) Angiosarcoma

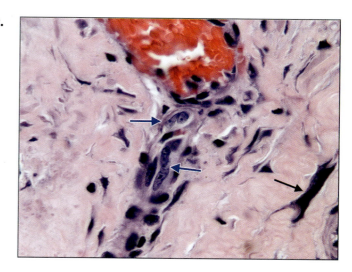

2. **A 55-year-old man has this 8 cm retroperitoneal mass. What karyotypic changes are most likely present?**
   - (a) Ring chromosomes
   - (b) Giant marker chromosomes
   - (c) Complex genetic changes
   - (d) No chromosomal changes
   - (e) Chromosome 16q aberrations

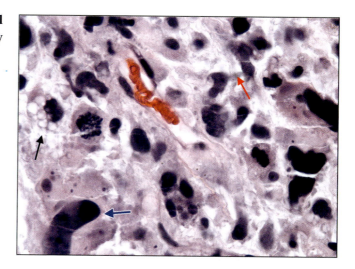

3. **Which of the following stains will reliably highlight this tumor?**
   (a) EMA
   (b) S-100
   (c) Pancytokeratin
   (d) CD34
   (e) None of the markers listed

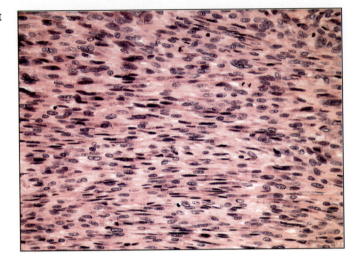

4. **A 58-year-old female has a 20 cm retroperitoneal mass. What is the most correct diagnosis?**
   (a) Osteosarcoma
   (b) Chondrosarcoma
   (c) Dedifferentiated liposarcoma
   (d) Rhabdomyosarcoma
   (e) Leiomyosarcoma

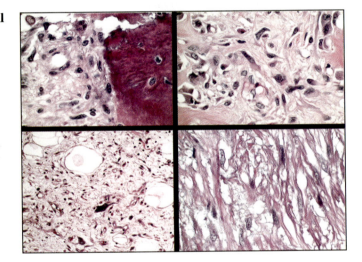

5. **Given the histology on the right of this left thigh lesion, what stain would support the diagnostic process?**
   (a) CD34
   (b) Actin
   (c) Desmin
   (d) S-100
   (e) Keratin

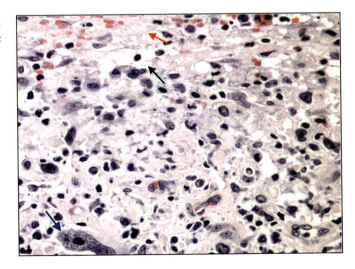

6. **An 87-year-old sun-damaged man with a history of squamous cell carcinoma of the scalp for which he was irradiated presents with a scalp lesion. What is the correct diagnosis?**
   - (a) Squamous cell carcinoma
   - (b) Basal cell carcinoma
   - (c) Atypical fibroxanthoma
   - (d) Pleomorphic liposarcoma
   - (e) Hodgkin's lymphoma

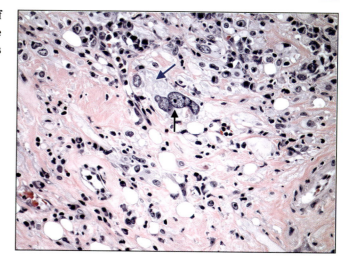

7. **A 70-year-old female has a 2.8 cm left calf mass that "just showed up one day". What is the correct diagnosis?**
   - (a) Pleomorphic liposarcoma
   - (b) Well-differentiated liposarcoma
   - (c) Undifferentiated pleomorphic sarcoma
   - (d) Dedifferentiated liposarcoma
   - (e) Pleomorphic lipoma

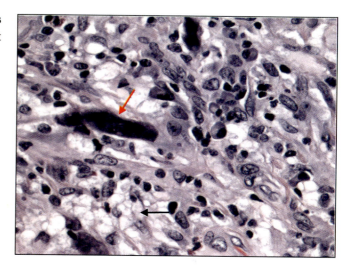

8. **Which two genes are most likely amplified in the tumor to the right?**
   - (a) Her2 and MDM2
   - (b) Her2 and CDK4
   - (c) CDK2 and MDM2
   - (d) CDK4 and MDM5
   - (e) MDM2 and CDK4

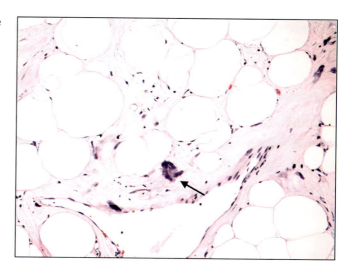

9. **Which of the following translocations is most likely found associated with this lesion?**
   (a) T(17;22)
   (b) T(7;16)
   (c) T(X;18)
   (d) T(12;22)
   (e) T(11;22)

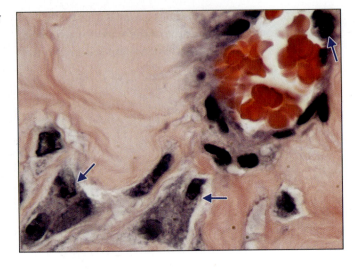

10. **What is the most likely site of metastases for the sarcoma depicted which stains negatively for CD34, desmin, FLT-1, and S-100?**
    (a) Lungs
    (b) Bone
    (c) Lymph nodes
    (d) Adrenal
    (e) Brain

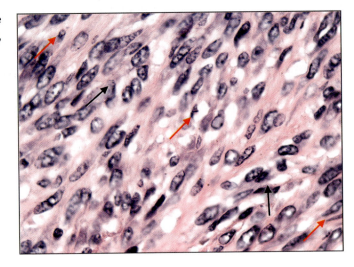

11. **A 59-year-old male has a 5 cm left forearm mass with heterogeneous T2 signal which is mostly intermuscular in position with minimal intramuscular extension. What is the most specific correct diagnosis?**
    (a) Inflammatory myofibroblastic tumor
    (b) Undifferentiated pleomorphic sarcoma, giant cell variant
    (c) Undifferentiated pleomorphic sarcoma, inflammatory variant
    (d) Undifferentiated pleomorphic sarcoma
    (e) Anaplastic large cell lymphoma

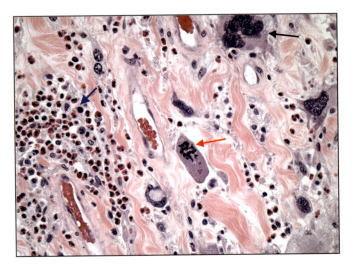

12. A 70-year-old man has a 10 cm mass near the right colon embedded in mature adipose tissue. What is the correct diagnosis?

  (a) Rhabdomyosarcoma

  (b) Spindle cell lipoma

  (c) Well-differentiated liposarcoma

  (d) Dedifferentiated liposarcoma

  (e) Pleomorphic liposarcoma

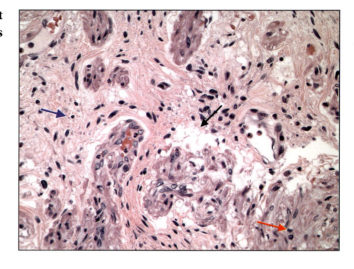

13. A 56-year-old man developed thigh pain and then a mass in the right lateral thigh. Imaging shows a 5 cm nontender mass in the right lateral thigh that just appeared one day, grew, then stopped growing. Imaging is nonspecific. What is the correct diagnosis?

  (a) Osteosarcoma

  (b) Nodular fasciitis

  (c) Fibromatosis

  (d) Undifferentiated pleomorphic sarcoma with a storiform pattern

  (e) Pleomorphic liposarcoma

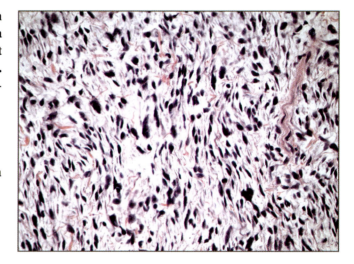

14. A 25-year-old male has the left ankle lesion depicted to the right. CD99 is positive and CD34 is negative. Which of the following stains would not stain these cells?

  (a) Cytokeratin

  (b) EMA

  (c) Bcl-2

  (d) TLE1

  (e) Chromogranin

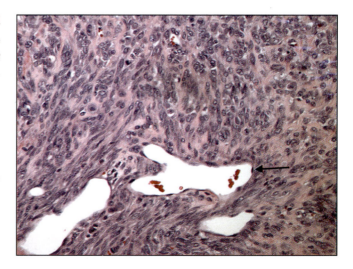

15. A 71-year-old has a large mass in the anterior lateral portion of the thigh. What is the correct diagnosis?
   (a) Pleomorphic liposarcoma
   (b) Atypical lipoma/well-differentiated liposarcoma
   (c) Pleomorphic lipoma
   (d) Spindle cell lipoma
   (e) Dedifferentiated liposarcoma

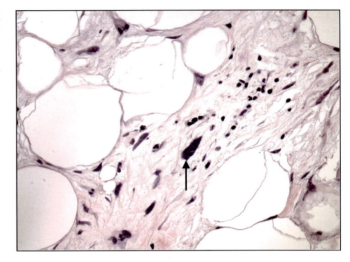

16. A 49-year-old female has a large soft tissue mass completely destroying the fibula in the mid to distal third of the fibula. CD99 and bcl-2 are positive in the tumor cells. CD34, smooth muscle actin, and S-100 are negative. What chromosomal rearrangement is most likely present?
   (a) T(11;22)
   (b) T(X;18)
   (c) T(X;17)
   (d) T(12;16)
   (e) T(17;22)

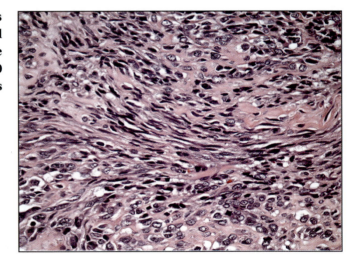

17. What clinical presentation is most often associated with this retroperitoneal tumor?
   (a) Dementia
   (b) Jaundice
   (c) Paraesthesias
   (d) Fever, leukocytosis
   (e) Hypercalcemia

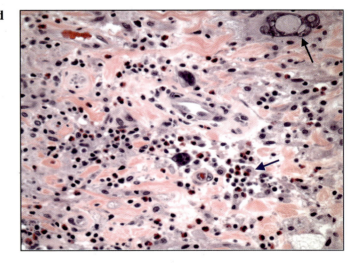

18. A 15-year-old girl has a heterogeneous enhancing 10.9 cm chest wall mass, with tumor invading the left pectoralis muscle and left axillary fat. There is cortical destruction of the left third, fourth, and fifth ribs. Histology from the mass is shown to the right and an S-100 stain is shown in the inset. Staining for smooth muscle, skeletal muscle, and melanoma markers are negative. A TLE1 stain is negative. What is the correct diagnosis?

    (a) Malignant peripheral nerve sheath tumor (MPNST)
    (b) Fibrosarcoma
    (c) Synovial sarcoma
    (d) Undifferentiated pleomorphic sarcoma
    (e) Leiomyosarcoma

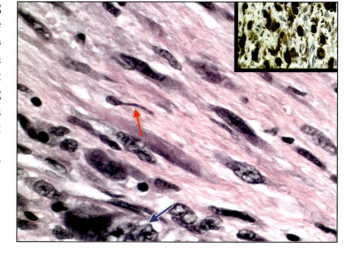

19. A 40-year-old female with a history of a left leg tumor status post chemotherapy now has a distal left femoral shaft lesion. What is the correct diagnosis?

    (a) Osteosarcoma
    (b) Stromal chemotherapy related atypia
    (c) Low-grade fibrosarcoma
    (d) Myxofibrosarcoma
    (e) High-grade fibrosarcoma

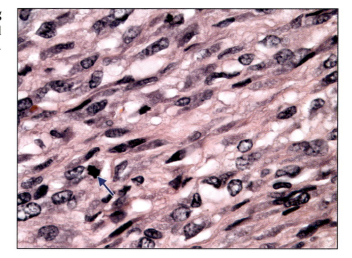

20. What is the most likely location for this lesion?

    (a) Thigh
    (b) Upper extremities
    (c) Abdominal wall
    (d) Scalp
    (e) Retroperitoneum

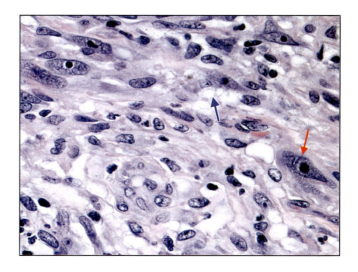

21. **A 73-year-old man presents with this scalp lesion. Which of the following is the strongest risk factor for this lesion?**
   (a) Previous trauma
   (b) Chemical exposure
   (c) Therapeutic radiation
   (d) HPV exposure
   (e) EBV exposure

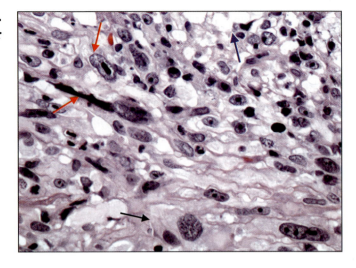

22. **A 27-year-old female has the lesion to the right excised that stains positively for desmin. In which of the following sites would this lesion be considered to have a high malignant potential?**
   (a) Deep thigh
   (b) Retroperitoneum
   (c) Uterus, submucosal
   (d) Uterus, subserosal
   (e) Cervix

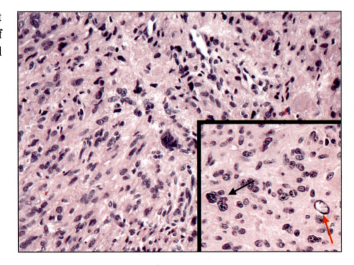

23. **A 26-year-old female has a 2.4 cm tumor in the right ethmoid sinus with right orbital and dural extension. Stains for smooth muscle actin and desmin are positive while a stain for caldesmon is negative. The correct diagnosis is:**
   (a) High grade fibrosarcoma
   (b) Monophasic synovial sarcoma
   (c) Storiform pattern undifferentiated pleomorphic sarcoma
   (d) High grade myofibroblastic sarcoma
   (e) Leiomyosarcoma

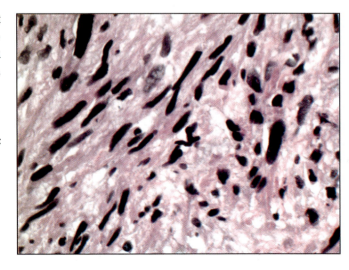

24. An 84-year-old female has a 8 cm left extremity mass with central necrosis extending into the soft tissue with high T2 signal. The lesion infiltrates the medial biceps and extends posteriorly to infiltrate the lateral and long heads of the triceps. What is the most correct diagnosis?
    (a) Undifferentiated pleomorphic sarcoma
    (b) High-grade myxofibrosarcoma
    (c) Low-grade myxofibrosarcoma
    (d) Pleomorphic liposarcoma
    (e) Undifferentiated pleomorphic sarcoma with giant cells

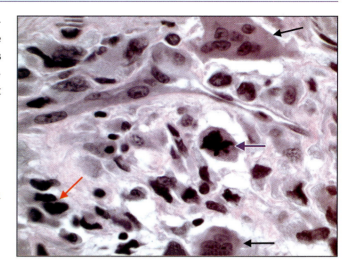

25. A patient has this tumor type in his lower extremity. The tumor cells stain negatively for cytokeratin, desmin, S-100, and myogenin. What is the approximate median 5 year survival for patients with this type of tumor.
    (a) 10%
    (b) 20%
    (c) 50%
    (d) 80%
    (e) 90%

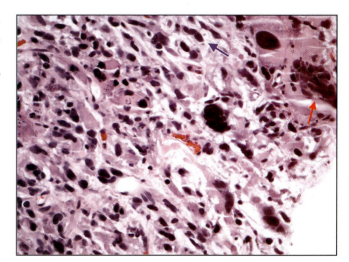

26. This 6 cm retroperitoneal mass in a 58-year-old female most likely represents a dedifferentiated
    (a) Liposarcoma
    (b) Chondrosarcoma
    (c) Osteosarcoma
    (d) No specific lineage
    (e) Rhabdomyosarcoma

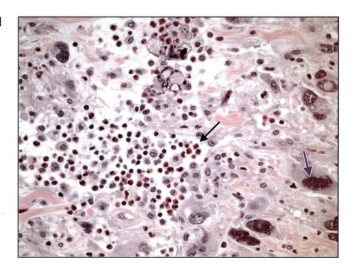

27. **A 65-year-old man with no known clinical history has the scalp lesion depicted. The neoplastic cells are negative for S-100 and pancytokeratin. What is the prognosis for this patient following resection?**
    (a) Poor
    (b) Intermediate
    (c) Variable
    (d) Excellent
    (e) Unknown

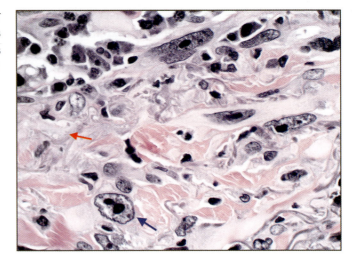

28. **What is the most common site for the depicted CD34 positive tumor?**
    (a) Skin
    (b) Liver
    (c) Soft tissue
    (d) Spleen
    (e) Bone

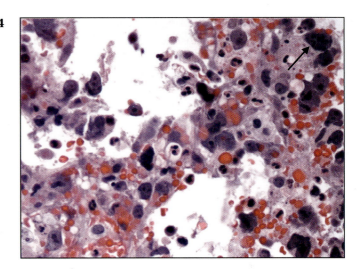

29. **A 68-year-old man has a right upper lobe lung nodule and a skin nodule. The cells are focally positive for S-100 but negative for HMB45, Melan-A, CD34, and desmin. What is the correct diagnosis?**
    (a) Clear cell sarcoma
    (b) Metastatic desmoplastic melanoma
    (c) Monophasic synovial sarcoma
    (d) Solitary fibrous tumor
    (e) Leiomyosarcoma

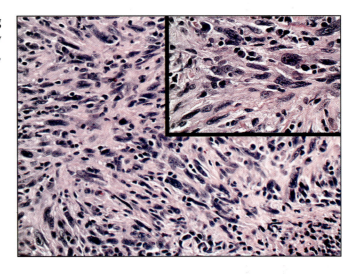

30. What cytogenetic abnormalities are most often associated with this tumor?

(a) Loss of 16q, 13q

(b) Complex multifocal changes

(c) Ring and giant marker chromosomes

(d) Ring chromosomes and complex multifocal changes

(e) T(12;22) and t(12;16)

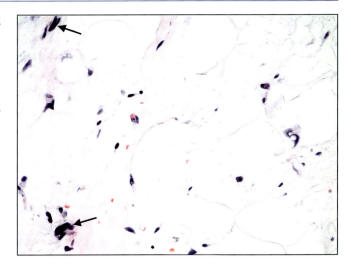

31. A 65-year-old man has a rapidly enlarging mass of the right thigh. What is the most likely karyotype?

(a) Complex karyotype

(b) PAX3-FOXO1A

(c) PAX7-FOXO1A

(d) 11p15.5 loss of heterozygosity

(e) No changes

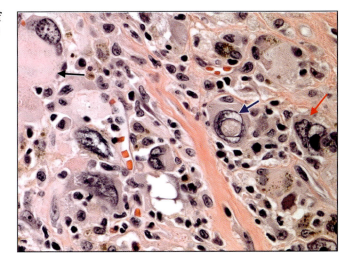

32. This retroperitoneal lesion in a 70-year-old man is associated with abundant mature adipose. What chromosomal pattern is most likely present?

(a) Loss of 16q, 13q

(b) Ring chromosomes and multifocal chromosomal abnormalities

(c) Multifocal chromosomal abnormalities without ring chromosomes

(d) No cytogenetic abnormalities

(e) Ring chromosomes and giant marker chromosomes

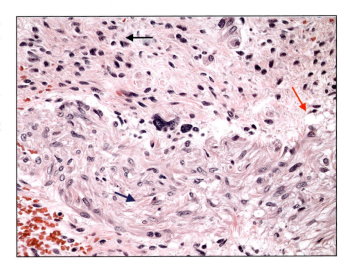

33. **A 63-year-old female has an 18 cm retroperitoneal mass that stains for desmin and exhibits high mitotic activity (>5/10 hpf). What is the correct diagnosis?**
    (a) Leiomyoma
    (b) Leiomyosarcoma
    (c) Dedifferentiated liposarcoma
    (d) Fibrosarcoma
    (e) Leiomyoma with degenerative atypia

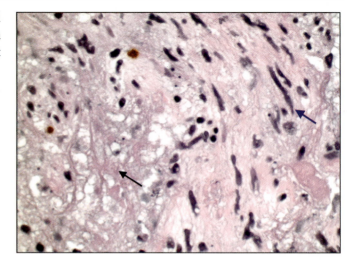

34. **A 75-year-old female has a slowly growing anterior left knee mass. Cytogenetic testing shows a TGFBR3-MGEA5 translocation. What is the correct diagnosis?**
    (a) Inflammatory myofibroblastic tumor
    (b) Myxoinflammatory fibroblastic sarcoma
    (c) Myxoid undifferentiated pleomorphic sarcoma
    (d) Inflammatory undifferentiated pleomorphic sarcoma
    (e) Giant cell undifferentiated pleomorphic sarcoma

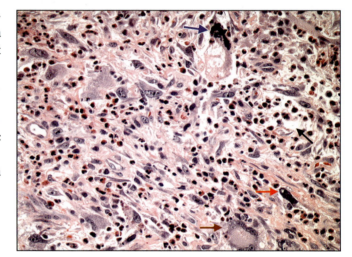

35. **A 76-year-old female has worsening dyspnea with anasarca. She has a 8 cm mass in the right atrium with possible involvement of the right ventricle. The comprehensive immunophenotype is nonspecific but cytogenetic testing reveals a SYT-SSX translocation. Which of the following is the correct diagnosis?**
    (a) Intimal sarcoma
    (b) Cardiac rhabdomyoma
    (c) Cardiac myxoma
    (d) Synovial sarcoma
    (e) Leiomyosarcoma

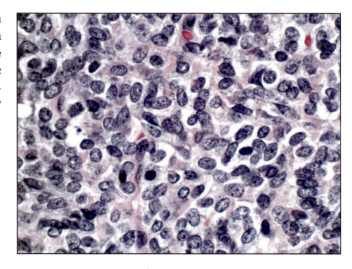

36. Which of the following karyotypic abnormalities is typical of this lesion?
(a) Ring chromosomes
(b) Giant marker chromosomes
(c) Loss of 16q and 13q
(d) Complex multifocal chromosomal changes
(e) No chromosomal changes

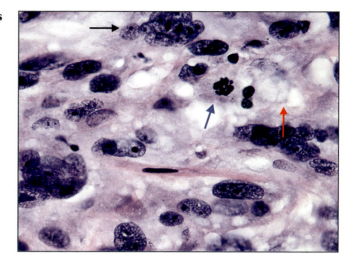

37. A 13-year-old girl has a 13 cm elbow mass, café au lait spots, and multiple additional smaller stable masses throughout her body. Histology from the elbow mass is shown to the right. What is the most likely site for metastases from her elbow lesion?
(a) Brain
(b) Lymph nodes
(c) Liver
(d) Lung
(e) Bone

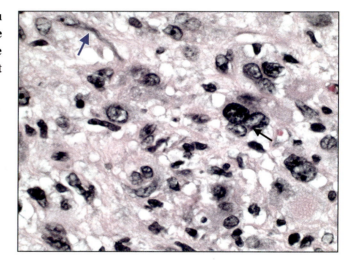

38. A 50-year-old man has an 8 cm posterior neck mass. What is the correct diagnosis?
(a) Lipoma
(b) Pleomorphic lipoma
(c) Hibernoma
(d) Angiolipoma
(e) Pleomorphic liposarcoma

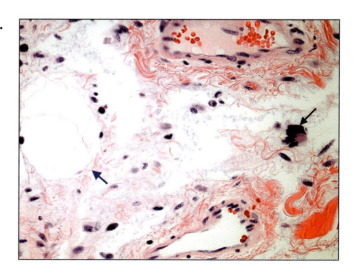

ANSWERS

1. **(c) Giant cell fibroblastoma**

   Giant cell fibroblastoma is a lesion characterized histologically by perivascular accumulations of multinucleated cells (blue arrows) and hyperchromatic cells (black arrow). The site is correct for elastofibroma but giant cells are not characteristic of it. More giant cells with a uniform distribution would be seen in giant cell tumor of soft parts. The cell highlighted by the black arrow would be consistent with chemotherapy atypia; however, perivascular accumulations of giant cells with otherwise bland appearing endothelial cells is not found in chemotherapy atypia. Angiosarcoma should show markedly atypical endothelial cells and a vascular proliferation; giant cells are not typically found in angiosarcoma.

2. **(c) Complex genetic changes**

   This case demonstrates severely atypical and hyperchromatic cells (blue arrow) admixed with myxoid areas (red arrow) and rare pseudolipoblasts (black arrow). Thus, the differential diagnosis includes pleomorphic liposarcoma, dedifferentiated liposarcoma, and undifferentiated pleomorphic sarcoma/ high grade myxofibrosarcoma. All three of these tumors display complex genetic changes. Ring chromsomes and giant marker chromosomes are found in well-differentiated liposarcoma and chromosome 16q aberrations are seen in spindle cell lipoma; neither of these lesions display sufficient atypia to be a diagnostic consideration.

3. **(e) None of the markers listed**

   The tumor depicted is a fibrosarcoma. The characteristic herringbone pattern can be appreciated and nuclear pleomorphism is present. CD99 would be positive in Ewing's sarcoma and synovial sarcoma. S-100 would highlight melanoma and some malignant peripheral nerve sheath tumors. Pancytokeratin would be positive in synovial sarcoma. CD34 would stain a GIST or vascular tumor. Fibrosarcomas rarely stain for these markers and most markers except for vimentin.

4. **(c) Dedifferentiated liposarcoma**

   This lesion demonstrates osteosarcomatous differentiation with osteoid formation by atypical cells (upper right), well-differentiated liposarcomatous differentiation (bottom left), and leiomyosarcomatous differentiation (bottom right). Dedifferentiated liposarcoma can dedifferentiate along multiple pathways including showing osteosarcomatous, angiosarcomatous, leiomyosarcomatous, and rhabdomyosarcomatous differentiation. Thus, tumors like this one that have multiple lines of differentiation and have a well-differentiated liposarcomatous component are most likely dedifferentiated liposarcomas.

5. **(d) S-100**

   The lesion shown is a pleomorphic liposarcoma which most commonly occurs in the thigh. Diagnostic features include bizarrely atypical meganucleolated cells (blue arrow), necrosis (red arrow), and multivacuolated lipoblastic cells (black arrow). Due to these features, pleomorphic liposarcoma is at the top of the differential diagnosis. Many cases of pleomorphic liposarcoma do not exhibit clear lipoblastic features and require an S-100 stain to highlight adipocytic differentiation. CD34, keratin, actin, and desmin have been reported to be positive in a fraction of pleomorphic liposarcomas but positivity in these cases would point away from the correct diagnosis.

6. **(c) Atypical fibroxanthoma**

   Atypical fibroxanthoma features a dermal population of severely atypical, bizarre cells (black arrow) embedded in a solar elastotic background (blue arrow). The presence of single atypical cells makes squamous cell and basal cell carcinoma less unlikely. The presence of solar elastosis, the clinical history of sun damage, and the site (scalp) are not consistent with Hodgkin's lymphoma or pleomorphic liposarcoma.

7. **(a) Pleomorphic liposarcoma**

   Pleomorphic liposarcoma features highly atypical cells (red arrow) with atypia in the spectrum of undifferentiated pleomorphic sarcoma and abundant polyvacuolated lipoblasts (black arrow). Without the presence of the lipoblasts, undifferentiated pleomorphic sarcoma would be correct. The cellularity is too high and the pleomorphism too great for a well-differentiated liposarcoma. In dedifferentiated liposarcoma we should also see a well-differentiated liposarcomatous area which is not present. Pleomorphic lipoma would demonstrate floret-type giant cells and not as much atypia.

8. **(e) MDM2 and CDK4**

The image depicts a well-differentiated liposarcoma with mature fat interspersed by atypical sparsely populated single cells (black arrow). Well-differentiated liposarcoma is characterized by amplification of MDM2 and CDK4. MDM2 and CDK4 both promote cell proliferation, the former by p53 inhibition and the latter through RB1 inhibition. These markers can help in the distinction of well-differentiated liposarcoma from lipoma in which they are not amplified.

9. **(a) T(17;22)**

This is a giant cell fibroblastoma. Proliferations of giant cells are seen in a perivascular distribution (blue arrows). T(17;22) is found both in giant cell fibroblastoma and dermatofibrosarcoma protuberans. T(7;16) is found in low grade fibromyxoid sarcoma. T(x;18) is characteristic of synovial sarcoma. T(12;22) is found in myxoid liposarcoma. T(11;22) is found in Ewing's sarcoma and desmoplastic small round blue cell tumor.

10. **(a) Lungs**

This is a fibrosarcoma, with a typical herringbone pattern. This pattern is highlighted by the arrows which show fascicles of malignant cells oriented in a repeating fashion, with fascicles marked with the red arrows giving an appearance of streaming in one way and fascicles highlighted by the black arrows appearing to stream in the opposite direction. The most common site of fibrosarcoma metastasis is the lungs followed by the bones. Hematogeneous spread is the rule and lymph node metastases are rare.

11. **(c) Undifferentiated pleomorphic sarcoma, inflammatory variant**

This lesion displays the main hallmarks of undifferentiated pleomorphic sarcoma, inflammatory variant: A significant mixed infiltrate of eosinophils and macrophages (blue arrow); markedly atypical cells (black arrow); and atypical mitoses (red arrow). Inflammatory myofibroblastic tumor would not show this degree of atypia. Undifferentiated pleomorphic sarcoma, giant cell variant, is not correct due to the lack of giant cells. In the absence of the inflammation, undifferentiated pleomorphic sarcoma would be the correct diagnosis; however, in this case, due to the prominent inflammation, undifferentiated pleomorphic sarcoma, inflammatory variant is more specific. Anaplastic large cell lymphoma should feature sheets of cells, not scattered atypical cells.

12. **(d) Dedifferentiated liposarcoma**

Dedifferentiated liposarcoma can take on two main forms, a form where the dedifferentiated areas are sharply demarcated from the well-differentiated areas, and another form where the two areas are intermixed, as in this image. The more well-differentiated areas with well-differentiated-liposarcoma-spectrum atypia and cellularity (blue arrow) make numerous interfaces with more spindled, pleomorphic, and cellular dedifferentiated regions (red arrow). The questions stem states that the lesion is embedded in mature adipose tissue and at the interface adipocytes can be seen, revealing the underlying differentiation of this lesion (black arrow). The retroperitoneum is the most likely site for this tumor.

13. **(d) Undifferentiated pleomorphic sarcoma with a storiform pattern**

The presentation of a lower extremity mass exhibiting sudden rapid growth is consistent with undifferentiated pleomorphic sarcoma. Histologically, these tumors contain severely atypical nuclei with hyperchromasia and high N:C ratios. Occasionally, as in this image, a spindled, vaguely storiform architecture can be present, leading to the modifier "with a storiform pattern". Undifferentiated pleomorphic sarcoma with a storiform pattern can cause diagnostic confusion with a high grade fibrosarcoma. The lack of osteoid rules out osteosarcoma. Nodular fasciitis and fibromatosis should not display the cellular atypia seen here. Furthermore, nodular fasciitis is seldom greater than 4 cm. Lipoblasts, seen in pleomorphic liposarcoma, are not present.

14. **(e) Chromogranin**

This is a monophasic synovial sarcoma with fascicles of spindled cells interspersed around hemangiopericytoma-like vessels (black arrow). Due to the CD34 negativity, hemangiopericytoma is unlikely and monophasic synovial sarcoma is the most likely diagnosis. Monophasic synovial sarcoma shows positivity for all the markers in the question except for chromogranin.

15. **(b) Atypical lipoma/well-differentiated liposarcoma**

The image depicts a well-differentiated liposarcoma. Among normal adipocytes are spindled cells some of which display significant atypia (black arrow). The atypia is not undifferentiated pleomorphic sarcoma-grade atypia and the lesion does not contain multiple polyvacuolated lipoblasts, both findings seen in pleomorphic liposarcoma. There are no floret type giant cells that would be seen in pleomorphic lipoma. The atypia is too great for a diagnosis of spindle cell lipoma. There is no worse differentiated component that would suggest a dedifferentiated liposarcoma.

16. **(b) T(X;18)**

This is a synovial sarcoma. The tumor cells are spindled and epithelioid. Staining for CD99 and bcl-2 moves synovial sarcoma and hemangiopericytoma to the top of the differential diagnosis. CD34 negativity makes synovial sarcoma the most likely diagnosis. Synovial sarcomas are characterized by the t(X;18) SYT-SSX translocation in 90% of cases and this case was positive for the translocation. T(11;22) is seen in desmoplastic small round blue cell tumor and Ewing's sarcoma. T(X;17) is seen in alveolar soft part sarcoma. T(12;16) is found in myxoid liposarcoma and angiomatoid fibrous histiocytoma. T(17;22) is found in DFSP which would stain positively for CD34.

17. **(d) Fever, leukocytosis**

This lesion is undifferentiated pleomorphic sarcoma, inflammatory variant, evidenced by the significant infiltrate of eosinophils and histiocytes (blue arrow) with scattered markedly atypical cells (black arrow). Undifferentiated pleomorphic sarcoma, inflammatory variant, patients frequently experience systemic symptoms such as fever, weight loss, and leukocytosis along with symptoms from the tumor itself.

18. **(a) Malignant peripheral nerve sheath tumor (MPNST)**

MPNST is a high grade sarcoma with marked cytologic atypia (blue arrow), buckled nuclei (red arrow, suggestive of neural differentiation), and variable S-100 staining (inset). The tumor cells can be spindled as in this case and many are associated with a neurofibroma. If a tumor that is suspicious for MPNST is not associated with a neurofibroma, a panel of stains must be performed to rule out other possibilities. Fibrosarcoma is usually S-100 negative. Synovial sarcoma should stain for TLE1. Leiomyosarcoma would be highlighted by smooth muscle markers. Undifferentiated pleomorphic sarcoma would not stain for S-100.

19. **(e) High grade fibrosarcoma**

Fibrosarcoma displays herringbone architecture as shown in the image as well as a high mitotic rate (blue arrow). This is not low grade fibrosarcoma because of the high mitotic rate, moderate nuclear atypia, and hypercellularity of the lesion without much interspersed collagen between atypical spindled cells. Many fibrosarcomas are associated with a history of trauma. The absence of osteoid formation rules out osteosarcoma. Chemotherapy related atypia in the stroma is typically individual stromal cells and would not lead to the spindled fascicular proliferation seen in the image. The lesion does not display enough myxoid stroma for a diagnosis of myxofibrosarcoma.

20. **(a) Thigh**

This is a pleomorphic liposarcoma. Adipocytic differentiation is seen by the presence of multivacuolated lipoblastic cells (blue arrow). The nuclear size varies greatly from one cell to the next with bizarre meganucleolated cells (red arrow), suggesting this is a high grade sarcoma. The top two differential diagnoses are thus pleomorphic liposarcoma and dedifferentiated liposarcoma. In dedifferentiated liposarcoma, found most commonly in the retroperitoneum, the high grade component is typically not adipocytic. Additionally, this lesion shows no better differentiated regions, thus this lesion is most likely a pleomorphic liposarcoma. Meganucleolated bizarre lipoblasts are a hallmark of pleomorphic liposarcoma. The most common site for this lesion is the thigh.

21. (c) Therapeutic radiation

This lesion is an atypical fibroxanthoma. Characteristic features include bizarre meganucleolated cells and hyperchromatic cells (red arrows), a solar elastotic background (black arrow), and clear cell cytoloplasmic changes (blue arrow). The main risk factors for atypical fibroxanthoma are therapeutic radiation and sun exposure.

22. (a) Deep thigh

This is a spindle cell lesion displaying scattered highly atypical cells (black arrow) and nuclear pseudoinclusions (red arrow). The nuclear and cytoplasmic features suggest this sarcoma has smooth muscle differentiation which is confirmed by desmin staining. In contrast to smooth muscle tumors in other locations, atypia indicates malignancy when found in smooth muscle tumors located deeply in the soft tissues. Atypia per se is not necessarily a sign of malignancy in the uterus or cervix (bizarre or symplastic leiomyoma) or in retroperitoneal lesions (degenerative atypia). Mitoses and necrosis may or may not be conspicuous in leiomyosarcoma.

23. (d) High grade myofibroblastic sarcoma

This tumor demonstrates a fascicular arrangement of spindled cells with pale pink cytoplasm and highly atypical hyperchromatic enlarged nuclei. These histologic findings and positive staining for desmin and smooth muscle actin while staining negative for caldesmon are typical of high grade myofibroblastic sarcoma. High grade fibrosarcoma, monophasic synovial sarcoma, and undifferentiated pleomorphic sarcoma would not stain for smooth muscle actin and desmin. Leiomyosarcoma would be highlighted by smooth muscle actin, desmin, and caldesmon. The caldesmon stain is critical for differentiating this lesion from leiomyosarcoma.

24. (e) Undifferentiated pleomorphic sarcoma with giant cells

This variant of undifferentiated pleomorphic sarcoma displays numerous multinucleated giant cells (black arrow), mitotic activity (blue arrow), and atypical hyperchromatic nuclei (red arrow). The numerous giant cells makes the other answer choices incorrect. This lesion has a similar prognosis to undifferentiated pleomorphic sarcoma.

25. (c) 50%

Considered a diagnosis of exclusion, in the face of severe cytologic atypia (red arrow), with no immunohistochemical evidence of differentiation, this tumor is a undifferentiated pleomorphic sarcoma. Some of these tumors can exhibit focally myxoid regions (blue arrow) leading some cases to be named high grade myxofibrosarcoma. The lower extremity is a typical site for this tumor. The median five year survival for undifferentiated pleomorphic sarcoma is approximately 50%.

26. (a) Liposarcoma

This is a undifferentiated pleomorphic sarcoma, inflammatory variant, as evidenced by a significant inflammatory infiltrate (black arrow) and scattered large atypical cells (blue arrow). Retroperitoneal undifferentiated pleomorphic sarcoma with inflammatory cells cases are almost uniformly synonymous with dedifferentiated liposarcomas due to the presence of chromosome 12q13-15 amplification and high levels of MDM2 expression in both groups.

27. (d) Excellent

The lesion is an atypical fibroxanthoma. The scalp location and the age of the patient support this diagnosis. Markedly atypical cells (blue arrow) with background solar elastosis (red arrow) are the hallmark of this lesion. Despite the high cytologic atypia, patients with this lesion that undergo excision with negative margins have an excellent prognosis. Lymph node metastases have been documented but they are rare.

28. (a) Skin

This is an angiosarcoma. CD34 positivity is nonspecific and can be seen in epithelioid sarcoma, dermatofibrosarcoma protuberans, solitary fibrous tumor, vascular tumors, as well as immature hematopoietic tumors. The histology depicted shows large atypical cells (black arrow), with high nuclear to cytoplasmic ratios, admixed with RBCs and surrounding vessels. These findings are diagnostic of angiosarcoma. The most common site for angiosarcoma is now the skin. Less common primary sites include the liver, soft tissue, spleen, and bone.

29. **(b) Metastatic desmoplastic melanoma**

Desmoplastic melanoma, as illustrated here, can be a diagnostic pitfall since the image shows markedly atypical cells in a spindled pattern, suggestive of sarcoma. Additionally, the staining pattern is not typical of conventional melanoma which should stain S-100 positive, HMB45 positive, and Melan-A positive. Nevertheless, this is a metastatic desmoplastic melanoma which displays a unique S-100 positive, HMB45 and Melan-A negative staining pattern. Clear cell sarcoma can show S-100 positivity but the cells would be more glycogenated than those seen in the image. Monophasic synovial sarcoma would be negative for S-100. Solitary fibrous tumor would be positive for CD34. Leiomyosarcoma would show desmin positivity. A possible differential diagnosis not listed could be a malignant peripheral nerve sheath tumor. In a patient with neurofibromatosis this immunohistologic profile coupled with the history of a skin lesion would raise more concern for malignant peripheral nerve sheath tumor.

30. **(c) Ring and giant marker chromosomes**

This is a well-differentiated liposarcoma. The image displays the typical histologic findings including mature adipocytes and scattered atypical hyperchromatic cells (black arrows). Well-differentiated liposarcoma is associated with ring chromosomes and giant marker chromosomes. Loss of 16q and 13q is associated with spindle cell lipoma which would not be consistent with the atypia present. Complex multifocal changes are seen in pleomorphic liposarcoma which would be more atypical than the lesion depicted here. Ring chromosomes and complex multifocal changes are characteristic of dedifferentiated liposarcoma but no dedifferentiated component is present. T(12;22) and t(12;16) are found in myxoid liposarcoma which would feature a delicate vascular networks that is not seen here.

31. **(a) Complex karyotype**

This is a pleomorphic rhabdomyosarcoma judging from the abundant eosinophilic cytoplasm with eccentric nuclei (black arrow) and high level of cytologic atypia. Two abnormalities commonly seen in pleomorphic rhabdomyosarcoma are nuclear pseudoinclusions (blue arrow) and nuclear molding (red arrow). Pleomorphic rhabdomyosarcoma has a complex karyotype. PAX3-FOXO1A and PAX7-FOXO1A translocations are seen in alveolar rhabdomyosarcoma. 11p15.5 loss of heterozygosity is seen in embryonal rhabdomyosarcoma. Both alveolar and embryonal rhabdomyosarcoma show less atypia than that seen here. This is a rare tumor with the general architecture and cytology of a pleomorphic undifferentiated sarcoma showing striated muscle differentiation.

32. **(b) Ring chromosomes and multifocal chromosomal abnormalities**

This is a dedifferentiated liposarcoma. The image shows a more well-differentiated-liposarcomatous area (black arrow) adjoining a more pleomorphic, cellular, spindled, and dedifferentiated area (blue arrow). The question stem mentions that this lesion is associated with abundant mature adipose tissue and adipocytes are at the junction (red arrow), supporting underlying lipomatous differentiation. The well-differentiated liposarcomatous areas should cytogenetically display ring chromosomes and giant marker chromosomes. However, the dedifferentiated portion should have a complex karyotype with multiple diverse cytogenetic changes. Thus, the karyotype should be mosaic, reflecting both the well-differentiated liposarcomatous areas (ring chromosomes) and the dedifferentiated areas (multifocal chromosomal abnormalities). Loss of 16q, 13q is associated with spindle cell lipoma. The other incorrect answer choices do not reflect the mosaic nature of the karyotype.

33. **(b) Leiomyosarcoma**

This lesion meets diagnostic criteria for a leiomyosarcoma with the presence of coagulative necrosis (black arrow), cellular atypia (blue arrow), and the stated high mitotic rate. With coagulative necrosis, simply the atypia or the mitotic rate would merit the diagnosis leiomyosarcoma. Leiomyoma would lack all three of these characteristics. Although the site is good for dedifferentiated liposarcoma, no well-differentiated liposarcoma component is seen. Fibrosarcoma would stain negatively for desmin. Leiomyoma with degenerative atypia can be seen in the retroperitoneum; however, the presence of coagulative necrosis is not consistent with that diagnosis.

34. **(b) Myxoinflammatory fibroblastic sarcoma**

Myxoinflammatory fibroblastic sarcoma is composed of myxoid areas (black arrow) which abut hyalinized areas. There are pleomorphic spindled tumor cells (red arrow) with a mixed inflammatory infiltrate. An atypical mitosis (blue arrow) can be seen in this case as well as touton-type giant cells (brown arrow) that can be associated with this lesion. Inflammatory myofibroblastic tumor is unlikely due to the cytologic atypia present. Undifferentiated pleomorphic sarcoma is a close differential as well as its giant cell and inflammatory subtypes due to the giant cells and inflammation that accompany severe atypia in this case. However, the presence of the TGFBR3-MGEA5 translocation that has been found in the majority of myxoinflammatory fibroblastic sarcomas and not documented in undifferentiated pleomorphic sarcoma makes myxoinflammatory fibroblastic sarcoma the correct diagnosis.

35. (d) Synovial sarcoma

Due to the presence of the translocation, this lesion is a synovial sarcoma and not an intimal sarcoma. This lesion contains epithelioid cells deposited in a collagenous matrix with no definite differentiation. A nonspecific comprehensive immunophenotype and the intracardiac location would favor an intimal sarcoma. However, positive testing for the SYT-SSX translocation in a immunohistochemically nonspecific tumor is sufficient to merit a diagnosis of synovial sarcoma. The other answer choices are not consistent with the cytogenetic and immunophenotypic findings.

36. (d) Complex multifocal chromosomal changes

This is a pleomorphic liposarcoma. Defining features include the highly atypical multinucleated cells (black arrow), high mitotic rate (blue arrow), and numerous multivacuolated lipoblastic cells (red arrow). Ring chromosomes and giant marker chromosomes are seen in well-differentiated liposarcoma. Loss of 16q and 13q is seen in spindle cell lipoma. Pleomorphic liposarcoma, consistent with its high grade sarcoma nature, exhibits a complex karyotype.

37. (d) Lung

This is a malignant peripheral nerve sheath tumor (MPNST) from the clinical history of neurofibromatosis 1 symptoms (café au lait spots, numerous smaller masses), high level of cytologic atypia, (black arrow), and buckled wavy nuclei (blue arrow). These tumors can take on a spindled herringbone appearance or a more epithelioid appearance as in this case and 25%–50% of tumors arise in the background of NF1. The most likely metastatic destination of MPNST tumors is the lung, where 66% of metastases travel. MPNST metastasizes to the lymph nodes in only 10% of cases. Liver, brain, and bone have metastatic deposits less often than the lung.

38. (b) Pleomorphic lipoma

This lesion contains mature adipocytes (blue arrow) and scattered atypical floret-like giant cells with eosinophilic cytoplasm and peripherally oriented nuclei (black arrow). Atypical floret-like giant cells are the hallmark of pleomorphic lipoma. Lipoma would not feature these atypical giant cells. Hibernoma would show more brown fat. Angiolipoma would feature vessels with intravascular thrombi. Pleomorphic liposarcoma would have far greater atypia.

CHAPTER 3

Benign Entities

1. **What is the most common site for this tumor?**
   - (a) Back of neck
   - (b) Scapula
   - (c) Foot
   - (d) Buttock
   - (e) Arm

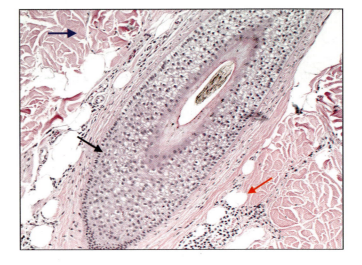

2. **An 86-year-old female with a history of metastatic ovarian cancer had a fall leading to a femoral fracture. Histology of the femur is shown. What is the correct diagnosis?**
   - (a) Metastatic carcinoma
   - (b) Osteopetrosis
   - (c) Osteopenia
   - (d) Benign bone
   - (e) Osteoarthritis

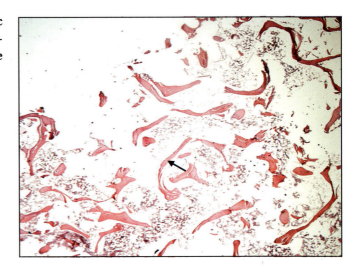

3. A 5-week-old product of a consanguinous union has pancytopenia. Shown is a bone marrow biopsy. What is the correct diagnosis?

  (a) Gaucher's disease
  (b) Osteoperosis
  (c) Osteopetrosis
  (d) Paget's disease
  (e) Normal bone

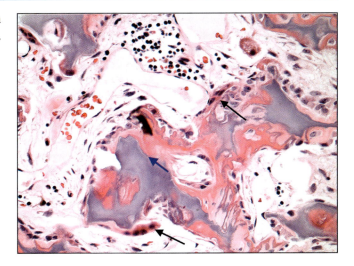

4. A 58-year-old female has an ill-defined enhancing 6 cm presacral mass which is worrisome for well-differentiated liposarcoma radiographically. What is the correct diagnosis?

  (a) Well-differentiated liposarcoma
  (b) Myelolipoma
  (c) Atypical lipoma
  (d) Spindle cell lipoma
  (e) Myolipoma

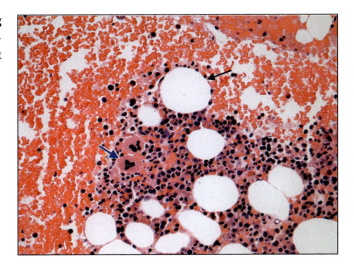

5. A 49-year-old diabetic female on hemodialysis missing one toe now has the second toe ulcer depicted to the right. What is the correct diagnosis?

  (a) Acute osteomyelitis
  (b) Chronic osteomyelitis
  (c) Multiple myeloma
  (d) Acute myeloid leukemia
  (e) Chronic myeloid leukemia

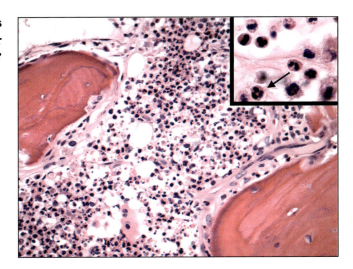

6. **A 45-year-old man presents with a posterior neck mass. What is the correct diagnosis?**
   (a) Elastofibroma
   (b) Fibromatosis
   (c) Gardner Fibroma
   (d) Nuchal type fibroma
   (e) Fibrolipoma

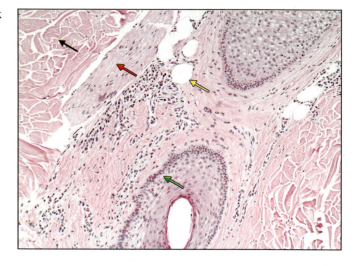

7. **A healthy 14-year-old boy fell on his arm but was able to keep playing football. A few days later while throwing a football he felt a snap in his arm followed by pain and distal numbness. Imaging showed a fracture. Two months later he noticed his arm becoming red and tender to the touch. The skin blistered, ruptured, and drained green fluid. Shown to the right is the humeral bone curettage specimen. What is the correct diagnosis?**
   (a) Normal bone marrow
   (b) Acute osteomyelitis
   (c) Chronic osteomyelitis
   (d) Langerhans cell histiocytosis
   (e) Sarcoidosis

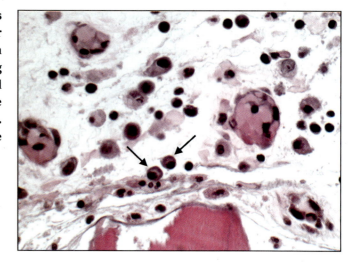

8. **What is the most common cause of this condition found during a woman's femoral arthroplasty operation for a fracture?**
   (a) Malnutrition
   (b) Old age
   (c) Chemotherapy
   (d) Corticosteroids
   (e) Homocystinuria

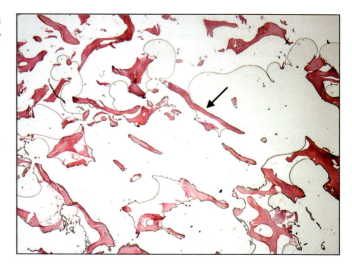

9. **An obese hypertensive 67-year-old man has a yellow lesion on his swollen great toe. What is the correct diagnosis?**
   - (a) Osteoarthritis
   - (b) Gout
   - (c) Rheumatoid arthritis
   - (d) Pseudogout
   - (e) Septic joint

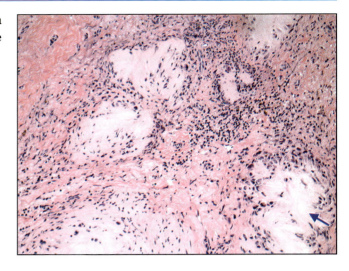

10. **A 74-year-old has moderate hand-joint pain and left shoulder joint pain. A humeral head arthroplasty operation yielded the histology to the right. What is the correct diagnosis?**
    - (a) Osteoarthritis
    - (b) Rheumatoid arthritis
    - (c) Gout
    - (d) Fracture callus
    - (e) Pseudogout

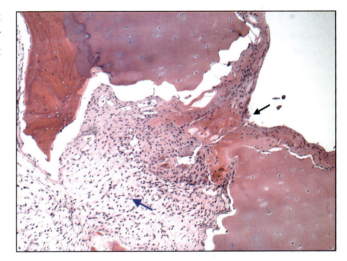

11. **A 48-year-old man has multiple masses distending the mid-ileum and projecting into the bowel lumen. What is the correct diagnosis?**
    - (a) Intestinal lipomatosis
    - (b) Hamartomatous polyps
    - (c) Tubular adenomas
    - (d) Hyperplastic polyps
    - (e) Normal bowel wall

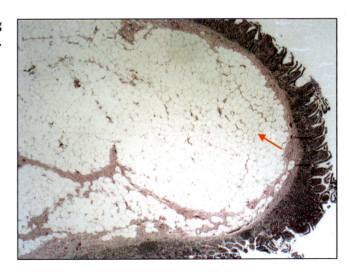

12. There is a 3.4 cm superficial soft tissue lesion in the upper back paraspinal muscles of a two year old boy. What gene is most likely mutated in this patient?

(a) von Hippel-Lindau (VHL)

(b) Tuberous sclerosis 1 (TSC1)

(c) Adenomatous polyposis coli (APC)

(d) Sodium channel, voltage gated, type V alpha subunit (SCN5A)

(e) Protein patched homolog 1 (PTCH1)

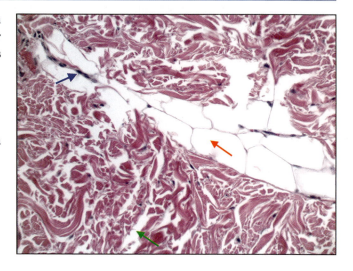

13. A 58-year-old woman with elbow pain and a history of symmetric joint pain has a left radial head arthroplasty operation. A representative from the arthroplasty specimen is seen to the right. What is the correct diagnosis?

(a) Septic arthritis

(b) Gout

(c) Pseudogout

(d) Rheumatoid arthritis

(e) Osteoarthritis

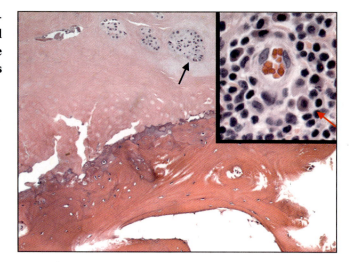

14. A 48-year-old man has a necrotic stage IV sacral decubitus ulcer. Imaging shows gas tracking into the right anterior thigh. Histology from a right upper leg skin excision is seen to the right. What is the correct diagnosis?

(a) Necrotizing fasciitis

(b) Proliferative myositis

(c) Polymyositis

(d) Dermatomyositis

(e) Inclusion body myositis

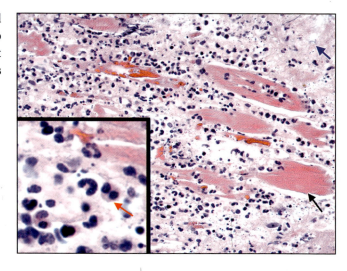

15. Which of the following is not a risk factor for the condition depicted?
   (a) Corticosteroid use
   (b) Vasculitis
   (c) Radiation
   (d) Vascular thrombosis
   (e) NSAID use

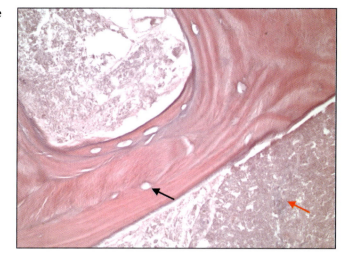

16. A 38-year-old female with a history of intravenous drug abuse has had ankle pain for 5 days. An excision from the capsule of the ankle joint near the distal tibia is shown to the right. What is the correct diagnosis?
   (a) Rheumatoid arthritis
   (b) Gout
   (c) Pseudogout
   (d) Septic arthritis
   (e) Osteoarthritis

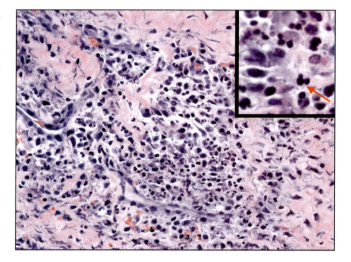

17. A 70-year-old female with knee pain has medial and lateral meniscus tears. A biopsy shows the histologic findings to the right. On high magnification, numerous structures seen in the inset are observed. What is the correct diagnosis?
   (a) Gout
   (b) Rheumatoid arthritis
   (c) Pseudogout
   (d) Osteonecrosis
   (e) Septic joint

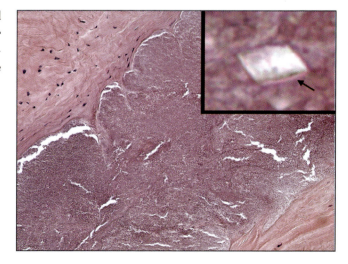

18. **Which clinical scenario is this 6 cm adrenal mass not associated with?**
    (a) Pheochromocytoma
    (b) Adrenal cortical adenoma
    (c) Conn syndrome
    (d) Tuberous sclerosis
    (e) Adrenal cortical hyperplasia

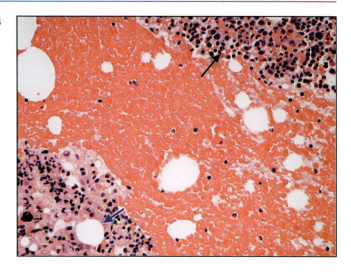

19. **A 23-month-old had a soft tissue mass on the right great toe that was excised once then recurred one year later. What is the correct diagnosis?**
    (a) Lipoma
    (b) Benign fibroadipose tissue
    (c) Lipoblastoma
    (d) Congenital fibrosarcoma
    (e) Fibrous hamartoma of infancy

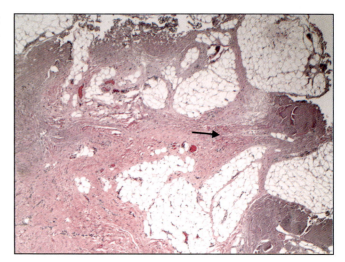

1. **(a) Back of neck**

   This is a nuchal type fibroma. Characteristic histologic features include dense fibrous tissue (blue arrow), entrapped adnexal structures (black arrow), and entrapped mature adipose tissue (red arrow). The most likely site of nuchal type fibromas is the back of the neck with far less common locations including the foot, buttock, and arm. Elastofibromas are found in the scapular region.

2. **(c) Osteopenia**

   Osteopenia, or osteoporosis, as shown in the image, contains markedly thinned bony trabeculae (black arrow) separating islands of normal trilineage hematopoiesis. Osteopetrosis would display osteocartilagenous trabeculae with activated osteoclasts. Metastatic carcinoma would show infiltrative nests of tumor cells. The trabeculae are too thinned for this to be normal bone; furthermore, the presence of normal bone does not explain the patient's femoral fracture which osteopenia does explain. Osteoarthritis features cartilaginous thinning, not bony trabecular thinning.

3. **(c) Osteopetrosis**

   Osteopetrosis shows irregularly shaped hybrid cartilaginous-osseous trabeculae (blue arrow) with prominent osteoclastic activity (black arrows). Infantile osteopetrosis is an autosomal recessive disease; thus, the clinical history of conasanguinity would predispose this patient to it. Gaucher's disease is also a recessively inherited disease; however, it would feature infiltration of the marrow by histiocytes. Osteoporosis is primarily a disease of the elderly and would feature thinned bony trabeculae. Paget's disease, like osteopetrosis, would show increased activity of osteoclasts; however, Paget's disease shows irregular cementum lines, not the osteocartilagenous septae seen in this case.

4. **(b) Myelolipoma**

   By definition, myelolipoma is a tumor that contains mature adipocytes (black arrow) and intermixed hematopoietic elements (blue arrow). None of the other lesions show hematopoietic elements.

5. **(a) Acute osteomyelitis**

   The history is a typical sequence of events involving end stage diabetics who are at risk for acute osteomyelitis. The patient is on dialysis for diabetic nephropathy and has had multiple toe ulcers due to diabetic neuropathy. The histologic image confirms acute osteomyelitis with the bone marrow packed with sheets of neutrophils (black arrow). Chronic osteomyelitis and multiple myeloma would not feature a prominent neutrophilic infiltrate. Given the clinical history, acute myeloid leukemia and chronic myeloid leukemia are unlikely.

6. **(d) Nuchal type fibroma**

   Dense fibrous tissue (black arrow) surrounds and entraps nerves (red arrow), mature adipocytes (yellow arrow), and hair follicles (green arrow). The back of the neck is the most common site for this tumor. Elastofibroma is found more commonly in the scapular region and does not feature entrapped adipocytes, adnexal structures, and nerves. Fibromatosis is more cellular and does not feature the dense collagen shown here. Gardner fibroma is a close differential; however, the age range is suboptimal for Gardner fibroma (a Gardner fibroma occurring over the age of 40 would be rare), while this patient is in the prime demographic for nuchal type fibroma (30 to 50 years of age). This amount of dense fibrous tissue with adnexal trapping is not seen in fibrolipoma.

7. **(c) Chronic osteomyelitis**

   This patient's curettage specimen shows multiple plasma cells (black arrows) which are the hallmark of chronic osteomyelitis. This proportion of plasma cells are not present in normal bone marrow. Acute osteomyelitis would show an abundance of neutrophils which are not present. Langerhans cell histiocytosis would show cells with grooved nuclei and eosinophilic inflammation. Sarcoidosis would show noncaseating granulomas.

8. **(b) Old age**

This is osteopenia, also known as osteoporosis, evidenced by the markedly thinned bony trabeculae (black arrow). The primary cause of osteopenia is old age, specifically the number of years after menopause, due to the increased bone resorption that occurs in women in the absence of estrogen. Malnutrition, chemotherapy, corticosteroid use, and homocystinuria are all less common causes of osteoporosis in women.

9. **(b) Gout**

Gout is associated with hypertension, obesity, and alcohol consumption. It occurs in adults and histologically features numerous nodules of amphophilic to eosinophilic feathery material lined by macrophages and giant cells (blue arrow). These nodules are named gouty tophi and are diagnostic of gout. Gouty tophi are a specific finding and are not found in the other answer choices.

10. **(a) Osteoarthritis**

Multifocal joint pain in an elderly individual raises concern for osteoarthritis. The histologic image shows the diagnostic findings of osteoarthritis including marked thinning and degeneration of the cartilage overlying the bone (black arrow) with associated granulation tissue (blue arrow). Rheumatoid arthritis would feature a more significant inflammatory infiltrate. Gout would show histiocyte-rimmed tophi and pseudogout would feature calcium pyrophosphate crystals. Fracture callus would have spindled cells as well as woven bone. The bone present here is degenerated mature bone.

11. **(a) Intestinal lipomatosis**

Several submucosal lobules (red arrow) composed of mature adipocytes are seen leading to bowel herniation into the lumen and obstruction. Large submucosal fat deposits are seen in intestinal lipomatosis but not in the other polyp types listed.

12. **(c) Adenomatous polyposis coli (APC)**

Depicted is a Gardner fibroma which features fat (red arrow) and vessels (blue arrow) entrapped by dense collagen. Spaces within the dense collagen can often be seen (green arrow), a phenomenon known as cracking. Gardner fibroma is associated with patients who carry mutations in the *APC* gene. VHL mutations lead to von Hippel Lindau syndrome, TSC1 mutations cause tuberous sclerosis, SCN5A mutations cause channelopathies, and PTCH1 mutations cause Gorlin syndrome, none of which are associated with Gardner fibroma.

13. **(d) Rheumatoid arthritis**

Rheumatoid arthritis typically affects middle aged women in their third to fifth decade. In this case, chondrocyte death is seen with only a few scattered islands of viable chondrocytes left (black arrow). The inset shows perivascular chronic inflammation (red arrow) that is typical of rheumatoid arthritis. Septic arthritis would show a prominent neutrophilic infiltrate. Gout would show macrophage-rimmed tophi. Pseudogout would show rhomboid crystals. Osteoarthritis would show chondral thinning and would not feature a prominent lymphocytic infiltrate.

14. **(a) Necrotizing fasciitis**

The image shows abundant necrosis (blue arrow) and necrotic myocytes (black arrow) infiltrated by florid acute inflammation (red arrow). The other answer choices would not include large amounts of acute inflammation and necrosis.

15. **(e) NSAID use**

This is osteonecrosis from the presence of necrotic adipocytes (red arrow) and empty lacunae (black arrow). Aseptic necrosis can cause fractures and has multiple possible etiologies. It can be due to corticosteroid use or vascular compromise in the form of vasculitis, radiation, or thrombosis. NSAID use has not been associated with the development of osteonecrosis.

16. **(d) Septic arthritis**

Septic arthritis features a large amount of neutrophils (red arrow) infiltrating synovial tissue, as seen in this image. Intravenous drug use is a risk factor for septic arthritis. Rheumatoid arthritis would show a lymphoplasmacytic infiltrate. Gout features tophaceous deposits lined by histiocytes. Pseudogout shows rhomboid crystals. Osteoarthritis shows degenerative changes without a significant inflammatory component.

17. (c) Pseudogout

Pseudogout typically involves the knee of an elderly (65–75 years old) patient. Histologically, numerous rhomboid shaped crystals are seen (black arrow) that weakly positively polarize. These crystals are deposited in a purple amorphous material and are composed of calcium pyrophosphate. In gout the crystals are needle shaped, negatively birefringent, and associated with histiocytes. Rhematoid arthritis and a septic joint would show significant inflammation that is not present. Osteonecrosis would show necrosis and dead bone which are not present.

18. (d) Tuberous sclerosis

This is a classical adrenal myelolipoma with hematopoietic elements (black arrow) and mature adipose tissue (blue arrow). These have been associated with certain clinical circumstances that lead to an overproduction of hormones including pheochromocytoma, adrenal cortical adenoma, Conn syndrome, and adrenal cortical hyperplasia. Tuberous sclerosis has not been associated with myelolipoma.

19. (c) Lipoblastoma

The image depicts a mature lipoblastoma. Lipoblastomas typically occur earlier than the age of three. The main histologic feature is lobules of fat separated by fibrous septae (black arrow). In lipoblastoma, the fat can have a range of maturity, from immature lipoblasts up to fully differentiated adipocytes as seen in this lesion. The key in the question stem that this may be a fully mature lipoblastoma is that it has been previously excised, suggesting that the lesion has longevity and has had time to mature fully. Lipoma is a good differential diagnoses; however, it does not show this classic lobulated adipocyte pattern. This could be mistaken for benign fibroadipose tissue without the history of a mass. Congenital fibrosarcoma would be more cellular. Fibrous hamartoma of infancy would show myofibroblastic fascicles and alcian blue positive regions which are not seen.

CHAPTER 4

Lesions with a Prominent Vascular Component

1. **A 32-year-old HIV-positive man has this lesion on his leg. What is the most likely etiologic agent?**
   (a) Staphylococcus aureus
   (b) HHV8
   (c) Bartonella Henselae
   (d) Streptococcus pneumonia
   (e) Bacillus anthrax

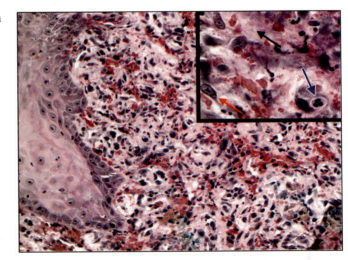

2. **A 35-year-old woman has a 2 cm subcutaneous mass on her right forearm. What is the correct diagnosis?**
   (a) Lipoma
   (b) Angiolipoma
   (c) Fibrolipoma
   (d) Spindle cell lipoma
   (e) Well-differentiated liposarcoma

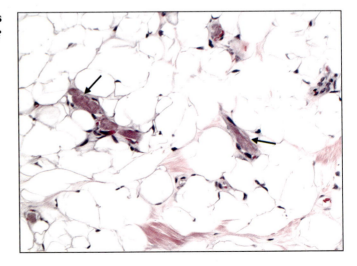

3. **A 30-year-old man has a right external ear lesion. The clinical suspicion is warts. What is the correct diagnosis?**
   - (a) Epithelioid hemangioendothelioma
   - (b) Epithelioid hemangioma
   - (c) Langerhans cell histiocytosis
   - (d) Granulation tissue
   - (e) Angiosarcoma

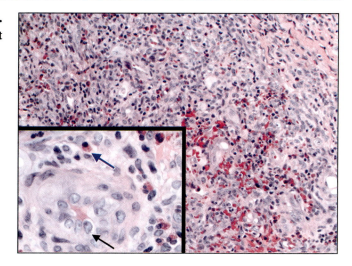

4. **A 14-year-old female with a history of angiosarcoma has a left inguinal crease nodule. What is the correct diagnosis?**
   - (a) Angiosarcoma
   - (b) Kaposi sarcoma
   - (c) Kaposiform hemangioendothelioma
   - (d) Spindle cell hemangioma
   - (e) Epithelioid hemangioendothelioma

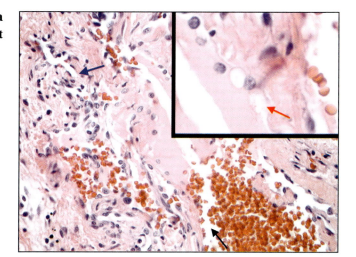

5. **A 10-year-old girl has a GLUT-1 negative pedunculated lower lip lesion. What is the correct diagnosis?**
   - (a) Juvenile capillary hemangioma
   - (b) Pyogenic granuloma
   - (c) Kaposiform hemangioendothelioma
   - (d) Angiomatosis
   - (e) Cherry angioma

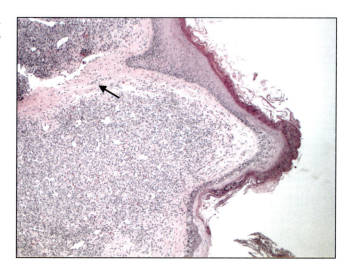

6. **A 53-year-old male has a left proximal tongue lesion. What is the correct diagnosis?**
   (a) Epithelioid hemangioma
   (b) Kaposiform hemangioendothelioma
   (c) Bacillary angiomatosis
   (d) Angiomatosis
   (e) Epithelioid hemangioendothelioma

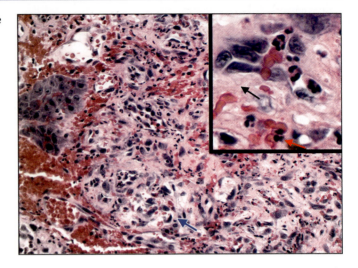

7. **A 52-year-old woman has a 6 cm liver lesion. The patient has no history of liver disease. What is the correct diagnosis?**
   (a) Angiosarcoma
   (b) Cavernous hemangioma
   (c) Lymphangioma
   (d) Kaposiform hemangioendothelioma
   (e) Epithelioid Hemangioendothelioma

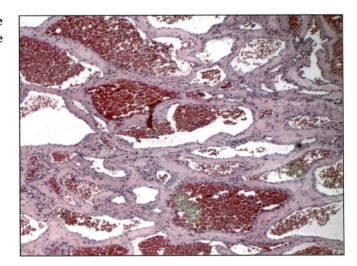

8. **The patient has had left knee articular complaints with joint catching for the past ten years. Imaging shows a synovial proliferation involving the left knee joint. A representative from the synovial lesion is shown here. What is the most specific correct diagnosis?**
   (a) Synovial hemangioma
   (b) Lymphangiomatosis
   (c) Angiomatosis
   (d) Cavernous hemangioma
   (e) Hemorrhage

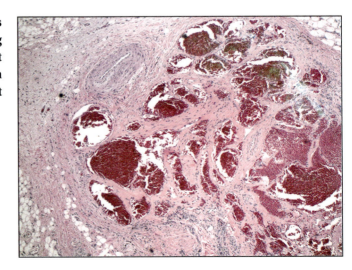

9. **What stain would have the highest chance of high-lighting this perivascular population of cells (blue arrow)?**
   (a) Smooth muscle actin
   (b) Pan-CK
   (c) HMB45
   (d) Synaptophysin
   (e) CD31

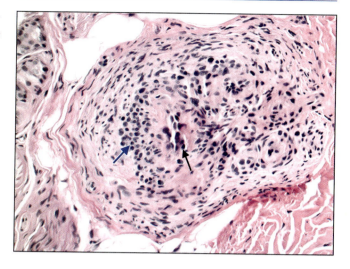

10. **A 10-month-old fair skin girl has a pink lesion on her right cheek. What stain can be used to distinguish this lesion from lobular capillary hemangioma?**
   (a) S-100
   (b) CD34
   (c) CD31
   (d) CK7
   (e) GLUT-1

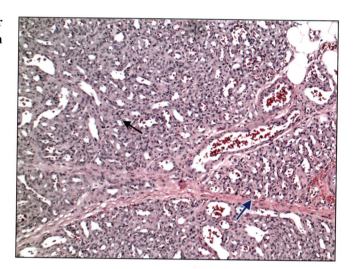

11. **A three-year-old male has multiple right upper arm and lung lesions with the histologic findings seen to the right. What is the correct diagnosis?**
   (a) Lymphangioma
   (b) Lymphangiomatosis
   (c) Angiosarcoma
   (d) Kaposiform hemangioendothelioma
   (e) Cavernous hemangioma

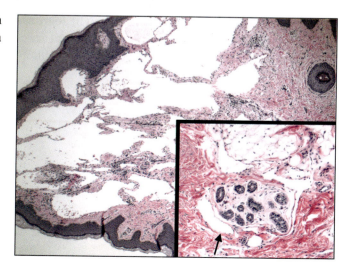

12. **A 44-year-old male has a 1 cm left alar rim intranasal mass. What is the correct diagnosis?**
    - (a) Angiofibroma
    - (b) Hemangioma
    - (c) Pyogenic granuloma
    - (d) Hemangiopericytoma
    - (e) Dermatofibroma

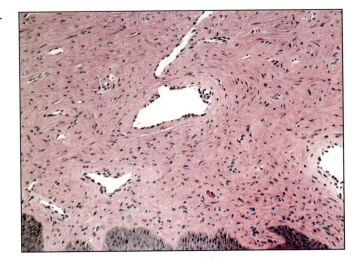

13. **This image was taken from a well-circumscribed mass in a 20-year-old male. What is the most likely site of this lesion?**
    - (a) Forearm
    - (b) Forehead
    - (c) Buttocks
    - (d) Retroperitoneum
    - (e) Abdominal wall

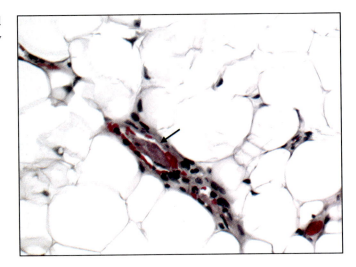

14. **The vulvar lesion depicted to the right features clusters of plasmacytoid cells radiating out from vessels on higher power. What stain is most likely positive in these cells?**
    - (a) ER
    - (b) S-100
    - (c) Pancytokeratin
    - (d) EMA
    - (e) CD34

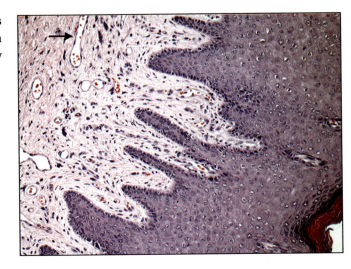

15. A 43-year-old woman has a slightly tender left cheek mass. What is the correct diagnosis?

(a) Pyogenic granuloma
(b) Angiomatosis
(c) Lymphangiomatosis
(d) Bacillary angiomatosis
(e) Angiosarcoma

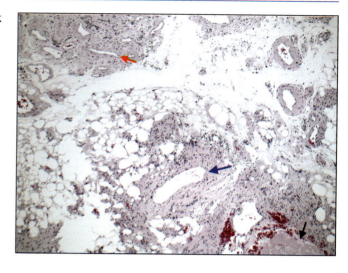

16. A 67-year-old has a right thigh mass. What is the correct diagnosis?

(a) Angiolipoma
(b) Myxoma
(c) Myxoid chondrosarcoma
(d) Myxoid liposarcoma
(e) Low grade myxofibrosarcoma

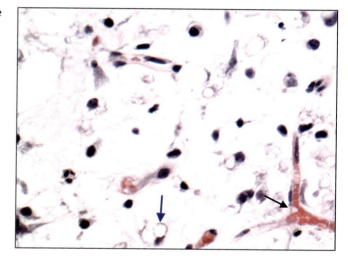

17. A 50-year-old man has a 6 cm anorectal junctional lesion. The clinical impression is lipoma. What is the correct diagnosis?

(a) Fibroma
(b) Cellular angiofibroma
(c) Angiolipoma
(d) Granulation tissue
(e) Spindle cell lipoma

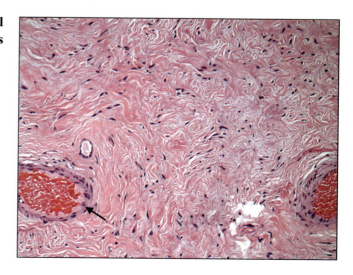

18. **A 39-year-old man has had a slowly growing left second toe soft tissue mass for the last few years which has caused deformity and ambulatory pain. What is the correct diagnosis?**
    (a) Leiomyoma
    (b) Angioleiomyoma
    (c) Hemangioma
    (d) Pyogenic granuloma
    (e) Fibromatosis

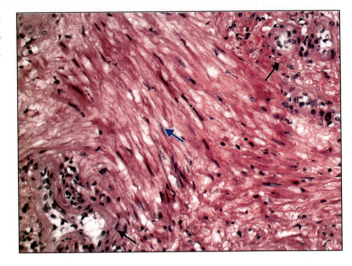

19. **A 65-year-old female has a left distal radius lytic lesion. Imaging shows an aggressive midshaft radial lesion, most likely metastatic disease or melanoma. Cortical bone destruction and periosteal new bone formation is present. Tumor cells stain positively for CD31. What is the correct diagnosis?**
    (a) Metastatic carcinoma
    (b) Pleomorphic liposarcoma
    (c) Epithelioid hemangioendothelioma
    (d) PEComa
    (e) Epithelioid hemangioma

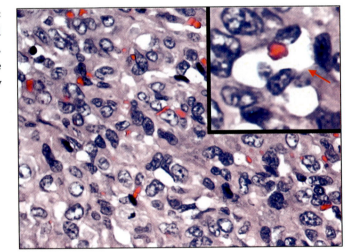

20. **What clinical scenario is most often associated with the depicted tumor?**
    (a) Osteoporosis
    (b) Osteomalacia
    (c) Gardner syndrome
    (d) NF2
    (e) Hypercalcemia

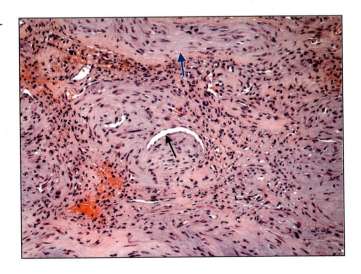

21. **A 9-year-old female has a 3 mm gingival nodule. What is the correct diagnosis?**
    (a) Cavernous hemangioma
    (b) Angiosarcoma
    (c) Lymphangioma
    (d) Pyogenic granuloma
    (e) Angiomatosis

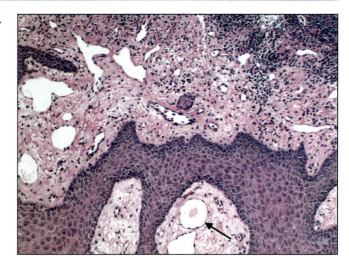

22. **Which of the following is the most significant risk factor for the tumor depicted?**
    (a) Smoking
    (b) Lymphedema
    (c) Foreign material insertion
    (d) Obesity
    (e) Alcohol

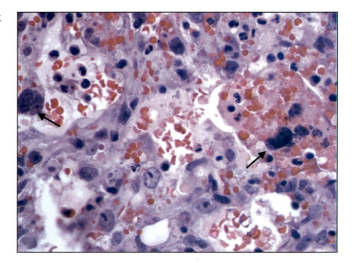

23. **A newborn has a vascular lesion involving the left paraspinal muscle and neighboring soft tissue. It is vimentin positive and Glut-1 negative. What syndrome is this newborn at greatest risk for?**
    (a) Birt-Hogg-Dubé syndrome
    (b) Kasabach-Merritt syndrome
    (c) Waterhouse-Friderichsen syndrome
    (d) Edward's syndrome
    (e) Sheehan's syndrome

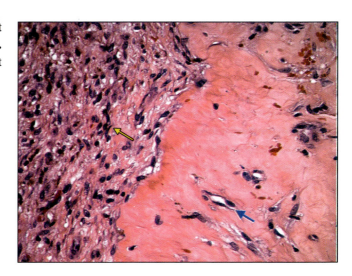

24. A 56-year-old has a 3 cm paracaval retroperitoneal mass abutting the duodenum and renal hilum. What is the correct diagnosis?
    (a) Angiomyolipoma
    (b) Myolipoma
    (c) Spindle cell lipoma
    (d) Angiolipoma
    (e) Well-differentiated liposarcoma

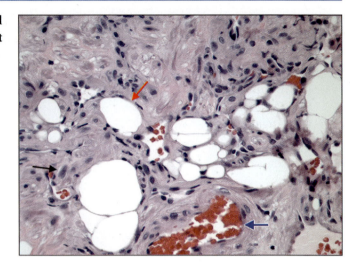

25. A 32-year-old Asian man has the 1.1 cm mass on his right neck depicted to the right. What describes the two top differential diagnoses?
    (a) Kimura disease vs epithelioid hemangioma
    (b) Kimura disease vs epithelioid hemangioendothelioma
    (c) Kikuchi disease vs epithelioid hemangioma
    (d) Kikuchi disease vs epithelioid hemangioendothelioma
    (e) Epithelioid hemangioma vs epithelioid hemangioendothelioma

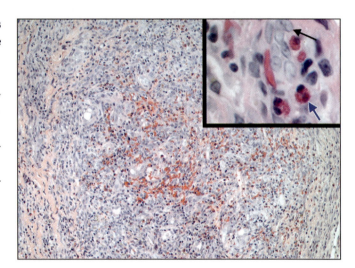

26. A 7-month-old has a superficial glabellar mass. What is the correct diagnosis?
    (a) Elastic hemangioma
    (b) Juvenile capillary hemangioma
    (c) Epithelioid hemangioma
    (d) Cavernous hemangioma
    (e) Cherry angioma

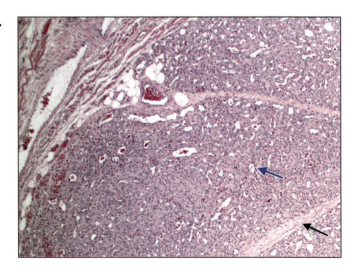

27. **A 55-year-old man has a large necrotic, hypodense, infiltrating, liver mass with abnormal LFTs and no history of liver disease. What is the most sensitive and specific antibody to label the tumor cells shown in the image?**
    (a) CD34
    (b) CD31
    (c) S-100
    (d) EMA
    (e) CK7

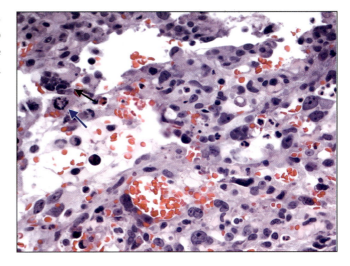

28. **A 6-month-old has a 2.5 cm ovoid scalp lesion which is heterogeneously enhancing. What is the correct diagnosis?**
    (a) Angiosarcoma
    (b) Kaposi's sarcoma
    (c) Intimal sarcoma
    (d) Papillary endothelial hyperplasia
    (e) Hemangioendothelioma

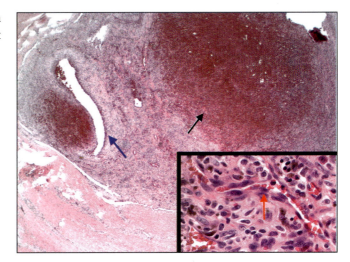

29. **A 66-year-old female has a 5 year history of a left anterior knee mass. The mass has grown larger and more tender in the past year. What is the correct diagnosis?**
    (a) Hemangiopericytoma
    (b) Myopericytoma
    (c) Synovial sarcoma
    (d) Glomus tumor
    (e) Myofibroma

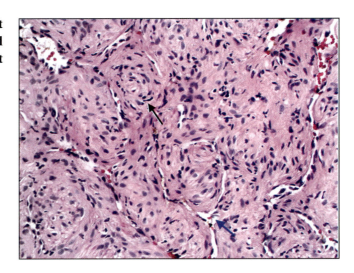

30. **A 12-year-old girl has a right arm lesion associated with pain and swelling. What is the correct diagnosis?**

(a) Angiomatosis

(b) Bacillary angiomatosis

(c) Pyogenic granuloma

(d) Angiosarcoma

(e) Cavernous hemangioma

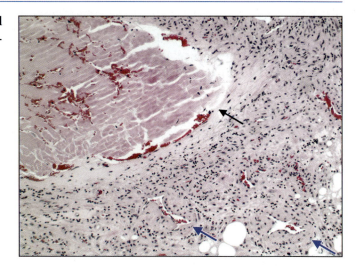

1. **(c) Bartonella Henselae**
   Given the history of HIV and the histologic findings, this is bacillary angiomatosis. Key histologic findings include a vaguely nodular pattern of plump endothelial cells (red arrow) with occasional cleared cytoplasm embedded in a pink fibrinous exudative matrix (black arrow). Bacillary angiomatosis also features an acute inflammatory infiltrate (blue arrow) that is seen in this case. Bacillary angiomatoisis is caused by members of the bartonella bacterial family. Given the clinical history, an important differential diagnosis is Kaposi sarcoma. However, this lesion does not display the classic spindling or slit like vasculature of Kaposi sarcoma.

2. **(b) Angiolipoma**
   Angiolipoma, as depicted in the image, contains mature adipocytes intermixed with a proliferation of capillaries, many of which contain fibrin thrombi (black arrows). This is a hypocellular angiolipoma. Lipoma would not contain the degree of vascular proliferation seen here. Fibrolipoma and spindle cell lipoma feature fibrous elements and spindled elements interspersed with the fat, respectively, not the capillary proliferation seen here. Well-differentiated liposarcoma would show more cytologic atypia or lipoblasts.

3. **(b) Epithelioid hemangioma**
   Epithelioid hemangioma, as seen in this case, is a vaguely nodular proliferation of capillary-sized vessels lined by bland endothelial cells, some of which project into the lumen, leading to a "tomb stone" appearance (black arrow). These lesions occur most often in the head and neck of young to middle aged adults. Most epithelioid hemangiomas also feature a brisk inflammatory infiltrate composed of eosinophils (blue arrow) and lymphocytes. In fact, another name for this lesion is angiolymphoid hyperplasia with eosinophilia due to the frequent finding of an eosinophilic infiltrate. Epithelioid hemangioendothelioma would show chords and strands of intracytoplasmically vacuolated cells in a myxoid or hyalinized stroma. Langerhans cell histiocytosis often features eosinophil rich infiltrates surrounding Langerhans cells, not capillaries. Granulation tissue would show vessel proliferation and inflammation; however, eosinophils do not predominate in granulation tissue. Angiosarcoma is unlikely due to the lack of hyperchromatic atypical nuclei.

4. **(d) Spindle cell hemangioma**
   This spindle cell hemangioma shows the typical findings of cavernous dilated blood-filled vessels (black arrow) surrounded by spindled cells embedding slit like vasculature (blue arrow). Some of the endothelial cells in the slitlike vasculature display a characteristic intracytoplasmic lumen (red arrow). Despite the slit like vasculature, angiosarcoma is unlikely due to the lack of cytologic atypia. Kaposiform hemangioendothelioma would show more spindling and cellularity. The histologic findings of small vessels surrounding a dilated vessel are suggestive of patch stage Kaposi's sarcoma; however, no inflammation is seen and such a lesion is unlikely in this age group. Epithelioid hemangioendothelioma contains cells with intracytoplasmic lumens; however, slit like and cavernous vessels are not characteristic of epithelioid hemangioendothelioma.

5. **(b) Pyogenic granuloma**
   This is a pyogenic granuloma with thick fibrous septae (black arrow) demarcating lobules of small capillaries. Juvenile capillary hemangioma is always a close differential with pyogenic granuloma; however, juvenile capillary hemangioma would have thinner fibrous septae and be GLUT-1 positive. Kaposiform hemangioendothelioma also can have nodules of capillary sized vessels but more solid spindled areas should be seen. Angiomatosis has irregularly shaped vessels with varying vessel caliber, neither of which is seen here. Cherry angioma has fewer capillaries per lesional area and features dilated often congested capillaries, not the small capillaries seen here.

6. **(c) Bacillary angiomatosis**
   The lesion depicted shows a vaguely nodular proliferation of plump endothelial cells embedded in pink fibrinous exudate (black arrow) with occasional cytoplasmic clearing (blue arrow), all findings seen in bacillary angiomatosis. An acute inflammatory infiltrate, one of the hallmarks of bacillary angiomatosis, is present (red arrow). Acute inflammation is not a prominent feature of the other answer choices.

7. **(b) Cavernous hemangioma**

This is a cavernous hemangioma with large dilated blood vessels filled with red blood cells and thick fibrous septae between blood vessels. Lymphangioma would show a proliferation of lymphatic channels, not blood vessels. No spindled cells or solid nodules are present which would be suggestive of kaposiform hemangioendothelioma. No myxoid or hyaline background is present to suggest epithelioid hemangioendothelioma. Angiosarcoma would feature irregular occasionally abortive blood vessels with cytologic atypia which are not seen.

8. **(a) Synovial hemangioma**

The synovial hemangioma depicted and described has large blood-filled vessels in a well-circumscribed nodule. Synovial hemangioma is histologically identical to cavernous hemangioma but occurs in the joint space and thus is the most specific correct answer. Lymphangiomatosis would not show blood-filled vessels. Angiomatosis would show vessels with varying sizes, not uniformly large dilated ones. Hemorrhage would not appear to be a proliferation of vessels.

9. **(a) Smooth muscle actin**

This is a glomus tumor with a proliferation of round monotonous cells with eosinophilic to amphophilic cytoplasm (blue arrow) encircling a blood vessel (black arrow). Glomus tumor cells are positive for smooth muscle actin and vimentin. They are usually negative for the remaining markers listed.

10. **(e) GLUT-1**

This is a juvenile capillary hemangioma. Diagnostic features include a proliferation of small vessels (black arrow) separated by fibrous strands (blue arrow). This lesion has considerable histologic overlap with lobular capillary hemangioma. Key differences are that lobular capillary hemangioma often is surrounded by an epidermal collarette and that juveline capillary hemangioma shows GLUT-1 staining while lobular capillary hemangioma does not.

11. **(b) Lymphangiomatosis**

Typical of lymphangiomatosis, this case shows a dermal proliferation of dilated channels which do not contain red blood cells. Also seen in lymphangiomatosis are lymphatic channels entrapping adnexal structures (black arrow). The multifocality of the disease merits the diagnosis of systemic lymphangiomatosis over lymphangioma. Angiosarcoma would show more atypia and slit-like vessels that are not seen. Kaposiform hemangioendothelioma would show solid nodules of spindled cells and a capillary proliferation. Cavernous hemangioma would feature a proliferation of dilated vessels filled with blood. The lung and bone are common sites of involvement by lymphangiomatosis.

12. **(a) Angiofibroma**

The angiofibroma depicted shows a proliferation of blood vessels, some of which are dilated and some of which exhibit irregular contours, suggestive of hemangiopericytoma vessels. There is a sparsely distributed population of spindled fibroblasts between the vessels with bland nuclear features. Irregularly shaped vessels and sparsely distributed fibroblasts are features of angiofibroma. Hemangioma and pyogenic granuloma would not have a spindled fibroblastic population between blood vessels. The spindled cell infiltrate between blood vessels in hemangiopericytoma is typically hypercellular and not sparse like that seen in this case. Dermatofibroma would show spindled cells but not the vascular proliferation seen here.

13. **(a) Forearm**

Angiolipoma, as depicted in the image, contains mature adipocytes intermixed with a proliferation of capillaries, many of which contain fibrin thrombi (black arrow). The most common site for angiolipoma is the forearm.

14. **(a) ER**

Angiomyofibroblastoma is characterized by a dermal proliferation of sometimes dilated vessels (black arrow) out of which radiate plasmacytoid, occasionally eosinophilic cells. An ER stain is diffusely positive in angiomyofibroblastoma. CD34 can show focal staining. The other markers are not expressed.

15. **(b) Angiomatosis**

Angiomatosis features numerous blood vessels of varying caliber occasionally with irregular shapes deposited in muscle or fat. Despite the relatively old age of the patient (most angiomatosis occurs before the age of twenty), large caliber (black arrow), medium caliber (blue arrow), and small caliber (red arrow) vessels are all represented in this image, making the correct diagnosis angiomatosis. Pyogenic granuloma would feature a proliferation of capillaries separated by fibrous bands. Lymphangiomatosis would show a proliferation of thin walled lymphatic channels, not blood vessels that contain a tunica media. Bacillary angiomatosis would show a proliferation of blood vessels with a significant amount of acute inflammation which is not seen here. Angiosarcoma would have cytologic atypia and slit like spaces.

16. **(d) Myxoid liposarcoma**

Myxoid liposarcoma is composed of spindled and vacuolated lipoblastic cells (blue arrow) deposited in a myxoid stroma with various cellularity. A characteristic finding shown here is the delicate vascular network of myxoid liposarcoma. Due to their intersecting and compressed appearance, these vessels are sometimes likened to crow's feet (black arrow). Angiolipoma, myxoma, myxoid chondrosarcoma, and low grade myxofibrosarcoma would not show lipoblasts.

17. **(b) Cellular angiofibroma**

As seen here, cellular angiofibroma contains blood vessels with thick hyalinized walls (black arrow) embedded in a stroma composed of randomly oriented short spindled cells. Fibroma and spindle cell lipoma would not have such prominent hyalinized vessels. Angiolipoma would feature non-hyalinized vessels with fibrin thrombi. Granulation tissue would have associated chronic inflammation.

18. **(b) Angioleiomyoma**

Angioleiomyoma is a painful lesion composed of a proliferation of blood vessels (black arrow) interspersed with fascicles of bland smooth muscle (blue arrow). Leiomyoma and fibromatosis would not feature such a proliferation of thick walled vessels seen here. Hemangioma and pyogenic granuloma would not have the well developed smooth muscle component.

19. **(c) Epithelioid hemangioendothelioma**

This epithelioid hemangioendothelioma shows sheets of epithelioid cells some of which contain intracytoplasmic lumens (red arrow) harboring red blood cells; the vascular differentiation of epithelioid hemangioendothelioma is at the unicellular level not the multicellular level found in most other vascular neoplasms. The epithelioid cells are often found in a myxoid or hyalinized stroma. Epithelioid hemangioendothelioma stains positively for vascular markers like CD31 and CD34. Metastatic carcinoma, pleomorphic liposarcoma, and PEComa will not contain intracytoplasmic lumens with red blood cells. Epithelioid hemangioma cells can show intracytoplasmic vacuoles; however, the lack of an eosinophilic infiltrate, the presence of the myxoid to hyaline stroma, and the presence of intracytoplasmic red blood cells make this diagnosis unlikely.

20. **(b) Osteomalacia**

This is a phosphaturic mesenchymal tumor. The basophilic chondromyxoid matrix (blue arrow) and the scattered irregularly shaped vessels (black arrow) are diagnostic features. This tumor is associated with oncogenic osteomalacia, with patients experiencing bone pain and atraumatic fractures.

21. **(c) Lymphangioma**

Lymphangioma shows a proliferation of dilated lymphatic channels (black arrow) with a thin lining in the dermis. Angiosarcoma would show more atypia. Cavernous hemangioma would show large, blood-filled vessels. Pyogenic granuloma would show an exuberant proliferation of capillaries in a lobular shape. Angiomatosis would show a variety of vessels of different sizes with occasional irregular shapes.

22. **(b) Lymphedema**

Blood-filled vascular spaces lined by highly atypical cells (black arrows) suggest angiosarcoma. Angiosarcoma is most commonly associated with radiation and lymphedema. Other less common associations proposed include foreign material insertion, either medically related, such as grafts, or material inserted related to an accident. No direct association with alcohol, smoking, or obesity has been reported yet.

23. **(b) Kasabach-Merritt syndrome**

This is a kaposiform hemangioendothelioma featuring capillary nodules some of which have a slit-like appearance (blue arrow) and more spindled regions reminiscent of Kaposi's sarcoma (yellow arrow). Over half of Kaposiform hemangioendothelioma cases are associated with Kasabach-Merritt syndrome, a clinical scenario featuring platelet consumption and thrombocytopenia which can be life threatening. Birt-Hogg-Dubé is associated with renal oncocytic neoplasms, Waterhouse-Friderichsen syndrome is associated with meningococcemia. Edward's syndrome is trisomy 18. Sheehan's syndrome is a pituitary infarct during pregnancy. A GLUT-1 stain was performed to rule out juvenile capillary hemangioma which should stain positively for GLUT-1 and also has a lobular arrangement of capillaries. Spindled cells are not a feature of juvenile capillary hemangioma.

24. **(a) Angiomyolipoma**

This image depicts the key histologic findings of angiomyolipoma: thick walled blood vessels (blue arrow); mature adipocytes (red arrow); and perivascular myoid cells (black arrow). Myolipoma is a close differential; however, the presence of thick walled blood vessels makes this diagnosis incorrect. Spindle cell lipoma and well-differentiated liposarcoma would not have a prominent vascular component. Angiolipoma would feature a proliferation of capillaries, not thick walled vessels, and it would have no perivascular myoid population.

25. **(a) Kimura disease vs epithelioid hemangioma**

This is an epithelioid hemangioma. Diagnostic features include a quasi-nodular architecture composed of capillary sized vessels with a prominent eosinophilic infiltrate (blue arrow) and bland endothelial cells (black arrow). A close differential diagnosis with epithelioid hemangioma is Kimura's disease which predominantly affects young Asian males, such as this patient. Kimura's disease features an eosinophil rich infiltrate along with lymphoid follicles and interfollicular vascular proliferation. If this were an interfollicular region from a Kimura lesion, the diagnosis instead could be Kimura disease. However, the absence of lymphoid follicles makes epithelioid hemangioma the most correct diagnosis. Epithelioid hemangioendothelioma would feature a myxoid or hyaline background and groups of cells with intracytoplasmic lumens; an eosinophilic infiltrate is not a feature of epithelioid hemangioendothelioma. Kikuchi disease is a necrotizing lymphadenitis that does not prominently feature eosinophils.

26. **(b) Juvenile capillary hemangioma**

Juvenile capillary hemangioma is characterized by lobules of small vessels (blue arrow) separated by fibrous strands (black arrow). Elastic hemangioma is associated with solar elastosis and is present in the elderly. Epithelioid hemangioma should feature a proliferation of epithelioid cells around vessels with an eosinophilic infiltrate which is not seen here. Cavernous hemangioma would have large, dilated, blood-filled vessels. Cherry angioma shows dilated, congested capillaries which are not seen here.

27. **(b) CD31**

This is an angiosarcoma from the proliferation of blood filled vessels lined by markedly atypical cells (black arrow) with occasional mitoses (blue arrow). CD34 and CD31 are diffusely positive in angiosarcoma. However, CD31 is more specific than CD34 since it does not highlight other soft tissue tumors such as solitary fibrous tumor, dermatofibrosarcoma protuberans, or epithelioid sarcoma. S-100 can be positive in angiosarcoma but is not as reliable as CD31 or CD34. EMA and CK7 are negative in most cases of angiosarcoma.

28. **(d) Papillary endothelial hyperplasia**

The image depicts thrombus formation (black arrow) with pseudovascular space formation (blue arrow), consistent with papillary endothelial hyperplasia. The cells that are creating the pseudovascular space, shown in the inset, are bland endothelial cells that can form slit like spaces (red arrow) suspicious for angiosarcoma. However, the absence of atypia, mitoses, and necrosis shows that this is not an angiosarcoma. Kaposi sarcoma would feature more of a spindled component associated with chronic inflammation. Intimal sarcoma would show more atypia. Hemangioendothelioma would show cells with an intracytoplasmic lumen.

29. **(b) Myopericytoma**

Myopericytomas typically contain irregularly shaped vessels (blue arrow) surrounded by a vaguely nodular (black arrow) proliferation of myoid-appearing cells. These cells have pink cytoplasm and a slightly spindled appearance, similar to the myoid cells of myofibroma. Hemangiopericytoma would not feature myoid nodules. Synovial sarcoma would have more cellularity and atypia. Though related to myopericytoma, glomus tumor would have epithelioid cells surrounding vessels without myoid nodules. Myofibroma would show myoid nodules without the irregular vascular pattern.

30. **(a) Angiomatosis**

Some cases of angiomatosis feature large dilated veins (black arrow) surrounded by smaller arterioles (blue arrows). Bacillary angiomatosis would show acute inflammation, pyogenic granuloma would show lobules, angiosarcoma would show atypia, and cavernous hemangioma would show uniformly dilated congested vessels.

CHAPTER 5

Lesions with a Prominent Myxoid Component

1. **What cytogenetic changes are most commonly associated with this lesion?**
   (a) t(12;16) and t(12;22)
   (b) Multifocal, complex changes
   (c) Ring chromosomes
   (d) Giant marker chromosomes
   (e) Loss of 13q, 16q

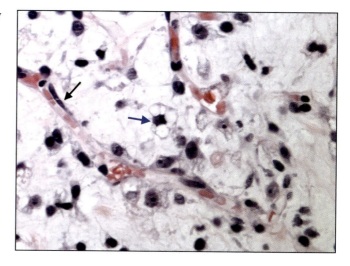

2. **A 55-year-old man has a 6 cm circumscribed deep upper arm mass. Histologically, there are thick fibrous septae separating lobules and each lobule has the histologic appearance shown to the right. What chromosomal translocation is most likely present?**
   (a) t(11;22)
   (b) t(9;22)
   (c) t(12;16)
   (d) t(7;16)
   (e) t(12;22)

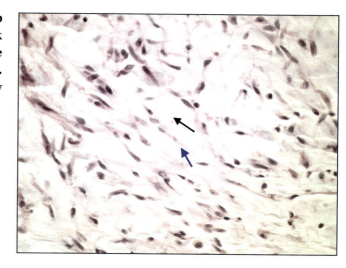

3. **A 42-year-old man has a 0.6 cm cyst on his third right toe. What is the correct diagnosis?**
   - (a) Dermal nerve sheath myxoma
   - (b) Myxofibrosarcoma
   - (c) Myxoid liposarcoma
   - (d) Cellular neurothekeoma
   - (e) Superficial angiomyxoma

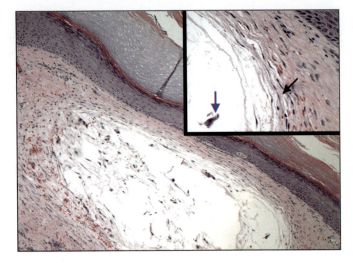

4. **A 59-year-old female has a lucent lesion of the anterior left iliac wing with no periosteal reaction. What is the correct diagnosis?**
   - (a) Chondroblastoma
   - (b) Chondroblastic osteosarcoma
   - (c) Chondromyxoid fibroma
   - (d) Chondrosarcoma
   - (e) Enchondroma

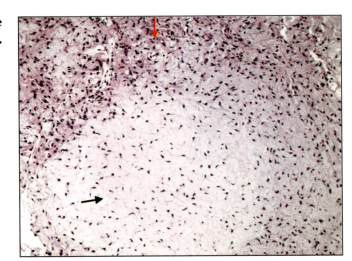

5. **What stain can be used to parse the top two differential diagnoses in this dermal skin lesion?**
   - (a) CD34
   - (b) Pancytokeratin
   - (c) Factor XIIIA
   - (d) C-Kit
   - (e) S-100

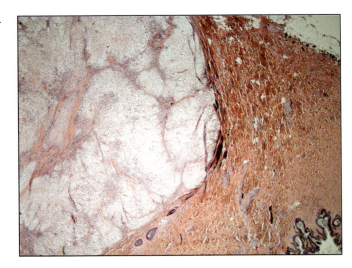

6. **A 33-year-old female has a slow growing well circumscribed encapsulated right distal thumb lesion that distorts the nail plate. Histology from the lesion is seen to the right. What is the correct diagnosis?**
   (a) Myxoid liposarcoma
   (b) Myxofibrosarcoma
   (c) Fibromyxosarcoma
   (d) Superficial acral fibromyxoma
   (e) Extraskeletal myxoid chondrosarcoma

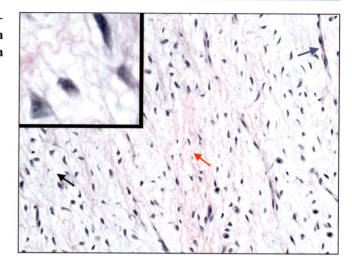

7. **A 56-year-old man has a left eyelid cyst. What is the correct diagnosis?**
   (a) Cutaneous angiomyxoma
   (b) Neurothekeoma/nerve sheath myxoma
   (c) Pyogenic granuloma
   (d) Aggressive angiomyxoma
   (e) Mucinous cyst

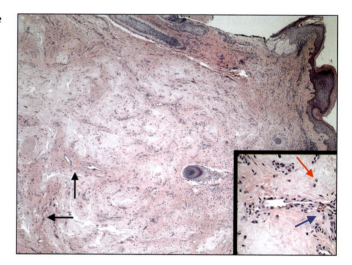

8. **A 9-year-old male has a 5 cm left lower quadrant abdominal dermal lesion. The preoperative diagnosis was pilomatricoma. An S-100 stain is negative. What is the correct diagnosis?**
   (a) Pilomatricoma
   (b) Dermatofibroma
   (c) Dermatofibrosarcoma protuberans
   (d) Myxoid neurothekeoma
   (e) Derman nerve sheath myxoma

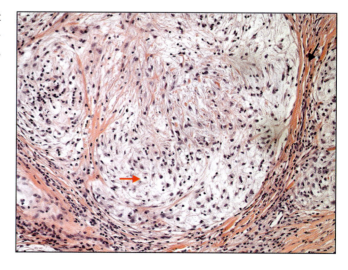

9. **A 36-year-old man has a 6 cm pleura-based mass extending through the neuroforamina into the epidural space with severe spinal cord compression. Most of the lesion has the appearance shown to the right, yet other regions display a myxoid hypocellular background with a network of delicate blood vessels. What is the most correct diagnosis?**
   (a) Myxoid liposarcoma
   (b) Myxoid chondrosarcoma
   (c) Ewing's sarcoma
   (d) Small cell carcinoma
   (e) Round cell liposarcoma

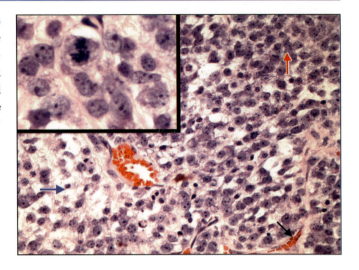

10. **A 31-year-old female has a 6 cm right mandibular mass associated with an unerupted tooth. What is the correct diagnosis?**
    (a) Myxoid liposarcoma
    (b) Extraskeletal myxoid chondrosarcoma
    (c) Odontogenic myxoma
    (d) Low grade myxofibrosarcoma
    (e) Fibromyxosarcoma

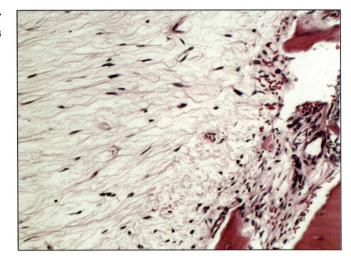

11. **A 74-year-old male has a 7.4 cm left upper arm mass. What is the correct diagnosis?**
    (a) Fibromyxosarcoma
    (b) Myxoma
    (c) Myxoid liposarcoma
    (d) Myxoid chondrosarcoma
    (e) Low grade myxofibrosarcoma

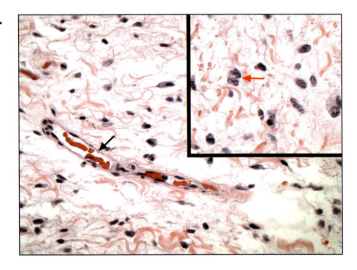

12. **A 43-year-old man was carrying heavy boxes at work until one day he developed a rapidly growing left thigh mass associated with pain. After its initial growth, the size of the mass plateaued and the pain decreased. What is the correct diagnosis?**
   (a) Pleomorphic liposarcoma
   (b) Low grade myxofibrosarcoma
   (c) High grade myxofibrosarcoma (undifferentiated pleomorphic sarcoma)
   (d) Fibromyxosarcoma
   (e) Fibrosarcoma

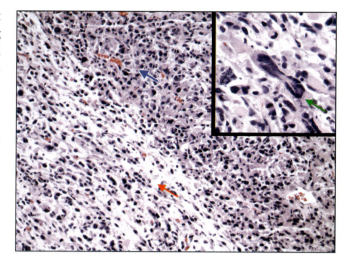

13. **A 41-year-old man has a 4.4 cm T2 hyperintense lobulated mass in the right fourth posterior rib at the costovertebral junction infiltrating the transverse process and compressing the T4 nerve root. Histology from the lesion is shown to the right. What is the correct diagnosis?**
   (a) Myxoid liposarcoma
   (b) Conventional intramedullary chondrosarcoma
   (c) Myxofibrosarcoma
   (d) Fibromyxosarcoma
   (e) Enchondroma

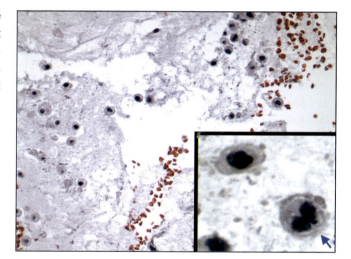

14. **A FISH test to identify this lesion would have to test for:**
   (a) T(12;16)
   (b) T(7;16)
   (c) T(6;9)
   (d) T(1;10)
   (e) T(11;22)

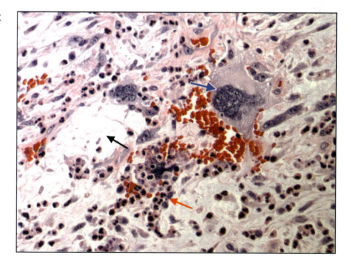

15. **A 64-year-old has a long history of a 9 cm right medial thigh soft tissue mass that is asymptomatic. What is the correct diagnosis?**
    - (a) Intramedullary conventional chondrosarcoma
    - (b) Myxofibrosarcoma
    - (c) Myxoid liposarcoma
    - (d) Intramuscular myxoma
    - (e) Extraskeletal myxoid chondrosarcoma

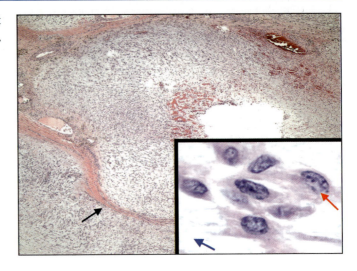

16. **What is the most common site for this radiographically well-defined tumor?**
    - (a) Lower extremities
    - (b) Upper extremities
    - (c) Retroperitoneal
    - (d) Scalp
    - (e) Scapula

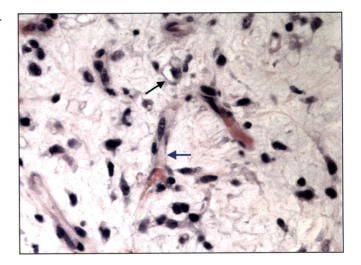

17. **A 59-year-old female has a 7.5 cm deep right ischiorectal fossa mass. Histology from the lesion is shown to the right. What is the correct diagnosis?**
    - (a) Cavernous hemangioma
    - (b) Angioleiomyoma
    - (c) Aggressive angiomyxoma
    - (d) Angiomatosis
    - (e) Angiomyofibroblastoma

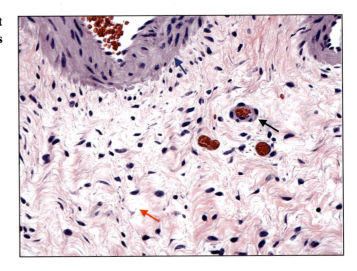

18. The widely metastatic lesion to the right has similar chromosomal changes to what tumor?
- (a) Myxoid liposarcoma
- (b) Pleomorphic liposarcoma
- (c) Myxofibrosarcoma
- (d) Pleomorphic undifferentiated sarcoma
- (e) Spindle cell lipoma

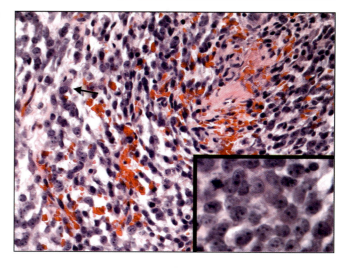

19. A 55-year-old female has a left knee soft tissue mass that clinically is thought to be a ganglion cyst. What is the correct diagnosis?
- (a) Ganglion cyst
- (b) Baker's cyst
- (c) Juxta-articular myxoma
- (d) Well-differentiated liposarcoma
- (e) Spindle cell lipoma

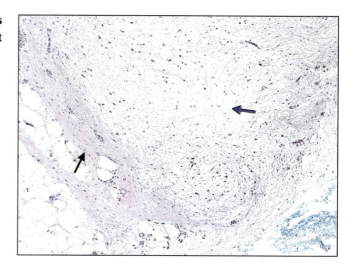

20. A 70-year-old female presents with a 2.5 cm soft tissue mass involving the right supraspinatus muscle. What is the correct diagnosis?
- (a) Myxoid liposarcoma
- (b) Low grade fibromyxosarcoma
- (c) Myxofibrosarcoma
- (d) Myxoid neurothekeoma
- (e) Myxoma

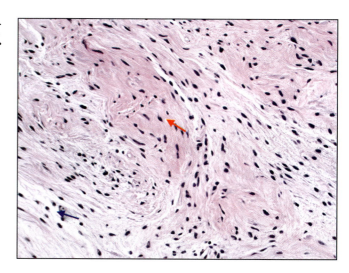

21. A 52-year-old man has a 17 cm multi-septated mass in the left gluteus muscle with an area of nondependent whorled contrast enhancement at the acetabular roof, worrisome for myxoid liposarcoma. What is the correct diagnosis?

   (a) Myxoid liposarcoma

   (b) Extraskeletal myxoid chondrosarcoma

   (c) Intramuscular myxoma

   (d) Myxofibrosarcoma

   (e) Fibromyxosarcoma

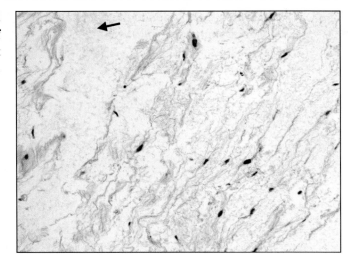

1. **(a) t(12;16) and t(12;22)**

   This is a myxoid liposarcoma with delicate compressed vasculature (black arrow) and lipoblasts (blue arrow) set in a myxoid stroma. T(12;16) and t(12;22) are the two most common translocations present in myxoid liposarcoma. Both of these translocations relocate the *DDIT3* gene. T(12;16) moves the gene to the FUS gene and t(12;22) moves it to the *EWS* gene. Multifocal, complex changes are found in pleomorphic liposarcoma which shows more atypia than that seen here. Ring and giant marker chromosomes are found in well-differentiated liposarcoma which does not typically have such a myxomatous background. Loss of 13q and 16q is found in spindle cell lipoma which has mature adipocytes, not lipoblasts.

2. **(b) t(9;22)**

   This is an extraskeletal myxoid chondrosarcoma. They occur in adults and are large tumors, most commonly arising in the proximal extremities. Histologically, they are composed of lobules of myxoid stroma separated by thick fibrous septae. As in the image, within this myxoid stroma (black arrow), spindled or epithelioid cords of cells (blue arrow) are seen. Extraskeletal myxoid chondrosarcoma has been associated with the t(9;22) translocation involving the *EWS* and *NR4A3* genes. T(11;22) is found in Ewing's sarcoma, a small round blue cell tumor. T(12;16) is found in myxoid liposarcoma which features prominent delicate vasculature. T(7;16) is characteristic of low grade fibromyxoid sarcoma which would show fibrous areas as well as myxoid areas. T(12;22) is seen in myxoid liposarcoma and clear cell sarcoma. Clear cell sarcoma would show greater cytologic atypia and cellularity without a myxoid matrix.

3. **(a) Dermal nerve sheath myxoma**

   Dermal nerve sheath myxoma is often found in the distal extremities. It is composed of nodules of spindled to stellate cells (blue arrow) deposited in a myxoid matrix. The nodules are surrounded by a thick fibrous capsule lined by wavy perineurial cells (black arrow). Lesions stain positively for S-100. Myxofibrosarcoma would display greater cytologic atypia. Myxoid liposarcoma would feature a delicate vascular network. Cellular neurothekeoma would have a higher density of cells and superficial angiomyxoma would have a more prominent vascular component.

4. **(c) Chondromyxoid fibroma**

   Chondromyxoid fibroma, depicted here, features hypocellular myxoid nodules (black arrow) and surrounding hypercellular fibrous regions (red arrow). Chondroblastoma and enchondroma do not feature hypocellular lobules like chondromyxoid fibroma. Chondroblastic osteosarcoma should show some osteoid deposition. Chondrosarcoma would show cartilage with a permeative infiltration of bone.

5. **(e) S-100**

   This is a myxoid neurothekeoma. The main diagnostic feature is a dermal proliferation of lobules containing cells deposited in a myxoid stroma. The architecture is not suggestive of carcinoma so pancytokeratin is not necessary. The lobulated nature of the lesion makes dermatofibroma (Factor XIIIA) and DFSP (CD34) unnecessary differential diagnoses to explore. Nerve sheath myxoma has very similar histologic appearance to myxoid areas of a neurothekeoma, both exhibiting a lobulated proliferation of edematous nodules containing bland spindled cells. S-100 is diffusely positive in nerve sheath myxoma and negative in neurothekeomas. C-kit would highlight a GIST which would not show the edematous stroma seen here.

6. **(d) Superficial acral fibromyxoma**

   Superficial acral fibromyxoma occurs in the hands and feet. The most commonly affected individuals are middle aged adults. Histologically, they are well-circumscribed lesions with myxoid (black arrow) to fibrous (red arrow) stroma in which sparsely distributed bland stellate to spindled cells are deposited. Also featured in the stroma of these lesions are prominent vessels with thin walls and a compressed appearance (blue arrow). Myxoid liposarcoma occurs in the deep soft tissues of the extremities and features lipoblasts which are not seen here. Myxofibrosarcoma would have more atypia. Fibromyxosarcoma is also found in deep soft tissues and would be predominantly fibrous. Extraskeletal myxoid chondrosarcoma should have cells in chords or chains, not haphazardly distributed. It is also found in the deep soft tissues and would feature thick fibrous septae dividing lobules.

7. **(a) Cutaneous angiomyxoma**

This lesion contains thick fibrous septae (black arrows) forming vaguely nodular myxoid regions. A network of delicate arborizing vessels (blue arrow) as well as discohesive single cells (red arrow) are distributed throughout the myxoid stroma. Neurothekeoma would be more definitively nodular and would not feature such a prominent vascular network. Pyogenic granuloma would not contain the myxoid regions. Aggressive angiomyxoma typically is a genital tumor arising most often in women. A mucinous cyst would not have a prominent vascular component.

8. **(d) Myxoid neurothekeoma**

Myxoid neurothekeomas features a circumscribed proliferation of nodular subunits containing bland splindled cells deposited in a myxoid matrix (red arrow). As in this question, neurothekeomas preferentially occur in young patients. The thick fibrous bands (black arrow) between individual myxoid lobules differentiate this lesion from pilomatricoma, dermatofibroma, and dermatofibrosarcoma protuberans. Myxofibrosarcoma would display more atypia than that seen here. Dermal nerve sheath myxoma can be histologically similar to myxoid areas of a neurothekeoma; however, it stains positively for S-100.

9. **(e) Round cell liposarcoma**

The question stem describes regions of myxoid liposarcoma elsewhere in the lesion. This specific image contains areas reminiscent of myxoid liposarcoma with curvilinear vessels (black arrow) and myxomatous patches (blue arrow). However, the tumor cells are round and the lesion is too cellular (red arrow) for a myxoid liposarcoma. Additionally, the tumor cells have prominent nucleoli and a high mitotic rate (*see* inset). This signifies that the tumor contains a round cell component, making it a round cell liposarcoma. When myxoid liposarcomas contain round cell liposarcoma areas, the prognosis is highly affected by the percentage of round cell component. This figure should be reported to the surgeon. Small cell carcinoma and Ewing's sarcoma have not been associated with myxoid liposarcoma. Myxoid chondrosarcoma would show fibrous septae separating lobules of cells with eosinophilic cytoplasm deposited in a myxoid stroma. No cells with eosinophilic cytoplasm or fibrous septae are present.

10. **(c) Odontogenic myxoma**

Typical of myxoma, the lesion displays bland haphazardly distributed stellate and spindled cells deposited in a myxoid background. Odontogenic myxomas typically occur in females in their second and third decades. The association with an unerupted tooth is also supportive of the diagnosis. Myxoid liposarcoma would have a delicate vascular network. Extraskeletal myxoid chondrosarcoma would show groups of cells deposited in a myxoid matrix with fibrous septae that are not seen here. Low grade myxofibrosarcoma and fibromyxosarcoma would show some fibrous regions.

11. **(e) Low grade myxofibrosarcoma**

Myxofibrosarcoma contains predominantly myxoid regions with few fibrous areas, as depicted in the image. High grade myxofibrosarcoma is synonymous with myxoid pleomorphic undifferentiated sarcoma which features bizarre malignant cells. Low grade myxofibrosarcoma, seen here, displays stellate and spindled cells deposited in a myxoid stroma with a low level of cytologic atypia, evidenced by binucleation (red arrow). The vasculature is often curvilinear (black arrow) but of a normal caliber, differentiating these vessels from the delicate vasculature of myxoid liposarcoma. Fibromyxosarcoma is unlikely since fibromyxosarcomas are more fibrous than myxoid. Myxoma should not exhibit binucleated tumor cells. Myxoid liposarcoma should be composed of lipoblasts and have a delicate plexiform vascular network. Myxoid chondrosarcoma should display fibrous septae between myxoid lobules and cells with eosinophilic cytoplasm which are not seen here.

12. **(c) High grade myxofibrosarcoma (undifferentiated pleomorphic sarcoma)**

This lesion displays myxoid areas (red arrow) next to more collagenous regions (blue arrow) along with bizarrely atypical cells (green arrow), all of which are features of high grade myxofibrosarcoma. The level of atypia rules out low grade myxofibrosarcoma and fibromyxosarcoma. Pleomorphic liposarcoma is not likely due to the lack of lipoblasts**.** Fibrosarcoma typically shows a herringbone pattern and does not have prominent myxoid regions.

13. **(b) Conventional intramedullary chondrosarcoma**

Conventional intramedullary chondrosarcoma can show mildly atypical (blue arrow) discohesive chondrocytes growing in a hyaline matrix or floating in a myxoid matrix, as seen here. The ribs is one of the most common sites affected by conventional chondrosarcoma. Despite the low grade nuclear features and the lack of architecture, the presence of chondrocytes in a myxoid matrix with aggressive radiologic features (bone infiltration and soft tissue involvement of the T4 nerve root) is diagnostic of conventional intramedullary chondrosarcoma. Myxoid liposarcoma would have more prominent vasculature and lipoblasts deposited in a myxoid matrix. Myxofibrosarcoma would show more atypia. Fibromyxosarcoma would have a prominent fibrous component. An enchondroma, particularly in the setting of Ollier's disease, could show this level of atypia; however, radiologic aggressiveness is not a feature of enchondroma. Additionally, enchondromas do not typically have a myxoid background.

14. **(d) T(1;10)**

This lesion contains highly atypical cells (blue arrow) deposited in a myxoid (black arrow)-hyalinized background and infiltrated by a dense mixed lymphoid population (red arrow), the hallmarks of myxoinflammatory fibroblastic sarcoma. This tumor is characterized by a t(1;10) translocation between TGFBR3 on chromosome 1 and MGEA5 on chromosome 10. T(12;16) is found in myxoid liposarcoma. T(7;16) is found in low grade fibromyxoid sarcoma. T(6;9) is characteristic of adenoid cystic carcinoma. T(11;22) is found in Ewing Sarcoma and desmoplastic small round blue cell tumor.

15. **(e) Extraskeletal myxoid chondrosarcoma**

Extraskeletal myxoid chondrosarcomas occur in adults and are large (most are greater than 5 cm). As in this case, the deep proximal extremities is the most common site for this tumor. Histologically, in extraskeletal myxoid chondrosarcoma, lobules of myxoid stroma are seen separated by thick fibrous bands (black arrow). The myxoid stroma (blue arrow) has bland epithelioid (red arrow) or spindled cells with eosinophilic cytoplasm arranged in groups (red arrow) or cords. No mature hyaline cartilage elements are seen in extraskeletal myxoid chondrosarcoma. Intramedullary conventional chondrosarcoma would not produce a soft tissue mass and prefers the central skeleton including the pelvis, ribs, and shoulder bones. Myxofibrosarcoma would show more atypia. Myxoid liposarcoma would have a prominent vascular component and vacuolated cells. Intramuscular myxoma contains sparsely distributed cells deposited in an abundant myxoid matrix. Having groups of cells, as in this case, would be atypical for myxoma.

16. **(a) Lower extremities**

This is a myxoid liposarcoma with delicate compressed appearing vessels (blue arrow) and lipoblasts (black arrow). The most common location for myxoid liposarcoma is the lower extremities.

17. **(c) Aggressive angiomyxoma**

This lesion is found in the genital region in middle aged and young adults. While more common in females, it can occur in males as well. Histologically, bland spindled cells are seen sparsely distributed in an edematous or myxoid stroma (red arrow). Also seen in the stroma are blood vessels some of which are thick walled (blue arrow) and some of which are thin walled (black arrow). Cavernous hemangioma would not have a spindled component and would contain all large dilated vessels. Angioleiomyoma would show streaming fascicles not haphazardly oriented cells. Angiomatosis would show large and small caliber vessels but would not show the edematous background or spindled cells seen in this lesion. Angiomyofibroblastoma most commonly involves the vulva but would not have a deep location and would not feature the large blood vessels depicted.

18. **(a) Myxoid liposarcoma**

This lesion is a round cell liposarcoma, as evidenced by the myxomatous regions (black arrow), monotonous round cells, and a vague streaming appearance. On high power a high mitotic rate and prominent nucleoli can be seen. Round cell liposarcomas are almost uniformly associated with myxoid liposarcoma-like regions and are thought to represent de-differentiated myxoid liposarcomas with a poorer prognosis. Consequently, they share the t(12;16) and occasional t(12;22) translocations.

19. (c) Juxta-articular myxoma

The image displays findings typical of juxta-articular myxoma: A sparsely populated spindled and stellate cell population is deposited in an edematous myxoid stroma (blue arrow). The nodule is encapsulated by a thick fibrous capsule (black arrow) in many cases of juxta-articular myxoma. Also, a pseudo-infiltrative appearance into nearby adipose tissue is seen in some cases of juxta-articular myxoma and can be seen here. Baker's cyst and ganglion cysts are true cysts without a myxoid region. Well-differentiated liposarcoma would not feature a large myxoid nodule and would show more atypia. Spindle cell lipoma would not feature myxoid nodules.

20. (b) Low grade fibromyxosarcoma

Low grade fibromyxosarcoma is characterized by fibrous regions with a proliferation of fibroblasts showing low nuclear grade (red arrow) adjoining myxoid areas (blue arrow) that contain bland spindled and stellate cells haphazardly distributed in an edematous stroma. The nuclei are regular with minimal cytologic atypia. The transition from myxoid to fibrous areas can be gradual or precipitous. Myxoid liposarcoma does not have the fibrous regions shown. Myxofibrosarcoma would show greater nuclear irregularity than what is seen here and has a greater myxoid component than fibrous component. Myxoid nodules in myxoid neurothekeoma have a septated quality that is not seen here. Myxomas do not have an accompanying fibrous element.

21. (c) Intramuscular myxoma

This tumor demonstrates bland haphazardly distributed spindled to stellate cells in a mucoid matrix with occasional cystic spaces (black arrow), which are all features of intramuscular myxoma. These lesions typically affect adults in the fifth to seventh decade of life. Myxoid liposarcoma would have more prominent vasculature. Extraskeletal myxoid chondrosarcoma would show groups of cells with eosinophilic cytoplasm. Myxofibrosarcoma would have more atypia and fibromyxosarcoma would display some fascicular architecture.

CHAPTER 6

Lesions with Epithelioid Cells or Abundant Vacuolated/Amphophilic/ Eosinophilic Cytoplasm

1. A 4-month-old has a 1.6 cm left ankle nodule with no bony invasion on imaging. Radiology believes it is consistent with a vascular malformation. CD68 and Factor XIIIA are positive while CD1a and CD117 are negative. What is the correct diagnosis?
   - (a) Myxoid liposarcoma
   - (b) Pleomorphic liposarcoma
   - (c) Juvenile xanthogranuloma
   - (d) Langerhans cell histiocytosis
   - (e) Mastocytosis

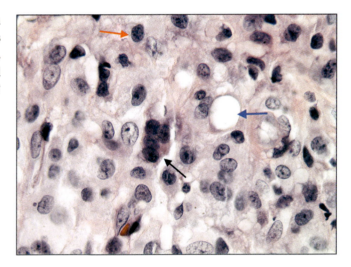

2. A 2-year-old boy has a 5 cm mass posterior to the bladder. Electron microscopic examination reveals compact aggregates of intermediate fibers with a vague whorling pattern. What is the correct diagnosis?
   - (a) Malignant extrarenal rhabdoid tumor
   - (b) Oncocytoma
   - (c) Granular cell tumor
   - (d) Eosinophilic variant of chromophobe renal cell carcinoma
   - (e) Multiple myeloma

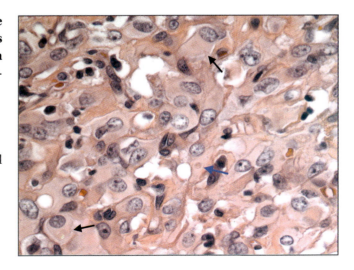

3. **A 75-year-old female with a history of a prior lesional excision in the esophagus now presents with recurrent disease in the larynx. What is the correct diagnosis?**
   (a) Adult rhabdomyoma
   (b) Granular cell tumor
   (c) Hibernoma
   (d) Fetal rhabdomyoma
   (e) Pleomorphic rhabdomyosarcoma

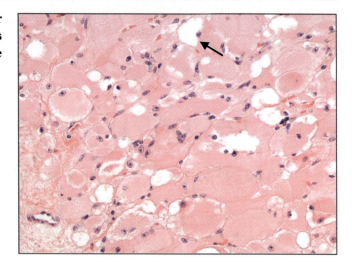

4. **Which immunohistologic pattern will be seen in this deep neck 3 cm soft tissue tumor from a 4-year-old boy?**
   (a) Negative staining for pancytokeratin
   (b) Positive staining for S100
   (c) Negative staining for vimentin
   (d) Negative staining for EMA
   (e) Loss of INI1

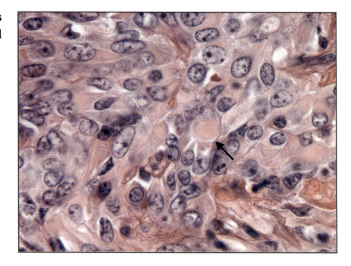

5. **A 33-year-old female has multiple pelvic osteolytic lesions radiographically concerning for metastatic disease. A biopsy of one lesion is shown here. What stain will least likely stain the tumor cells?**
   (a) EMA
   (b) Fli-1
   (c) CD31
   (d) CD34
   (e) CK7

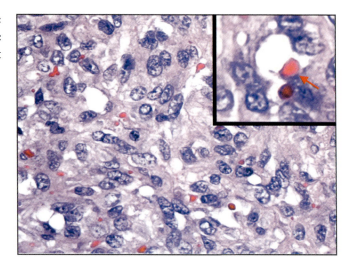

6. **A 39-year-old man has bilaterally enlarged lacrimal glands. What is the correct diagnosis?**
   (a) Signet ring cell carcinoma
   (b) Xanthoma
   (c) Tuberous xanthoma
   (d) Hibernoma
   (e) Verruciform xanthoma

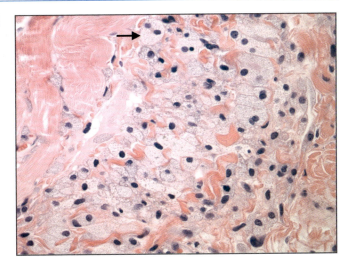

7. **A 31-year-old male has a 12 cm mass between the anterior and medial compartments of the superior thigh. The mass displaces but does not involve adjacent muscle. What is the correct diagnosis?**
   (a) Lipoma
   (b) Granular cell tumor
   (c) Hibernoma
   (d) Atypical lipoma
   (e) Spindle cell lipoma

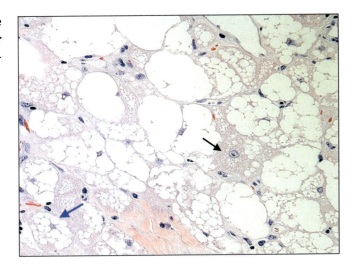

8. **A 15-year-old girl has a circumscribed 2.5 cm nodule on her right inner arm. The nodule has a hemorrhagic cut surface and the tumor cells stain positively for desmin. What is the most common translocation found associated with this lesion?**
   (a) T(2;22)
   (b) T(12;16)
   (c) T(12;22)
   (d) T(11;22)
   (e) T(X;17)

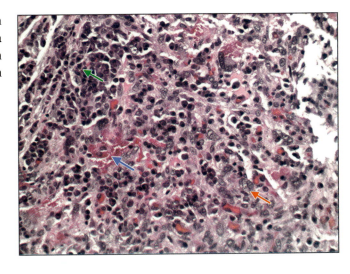

9. **A 14-year-old female has a small bowel mass. The radiologic differential was GIST versus leiomyoma. The tumor cells are negative for desmin. What is the correct diagnosis?**
   - (a) Desmoplastic fibroblastoma
   - (b) Leiomyoma with degenerative changes
   - (c) Calcifying fibrous tumor
   - (d) Metastatic lobular breast carcinoma
   - (e) Plexiform fibromyxoma

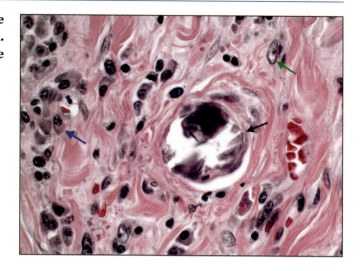

10. **An 18-year-old female has a right hip lesion. What is the correct diagnosis?**
    - (a) Tuberculosis
    - (b) Plexiform fibrohistiocytic tumor
    - (c) Granuloma annulare
    - (d) Epithelioid sarcoma
    - (e) Sarcoidosis

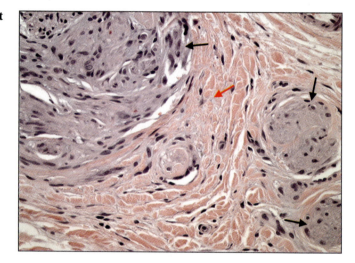

11. **A 59-year-old man has a 4 cm left dorsal hand soft tissue mass. A cytokeratin stain is positive and INI1 is lost in the nodular cells. What is the correct diagnosis?**
    - (a) Necrobiosis lipoidica
    - (b) Granuloma annulare
    - (c) Epithelioid sarcoma
    - (d) Miliary tuberculosis
    - (e) Infarction

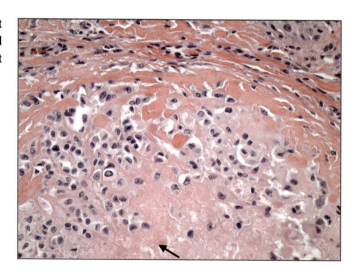

12. A 30-year-old male has a soft tissue mass of the right calf. Stains for HMB45 and Melan-A are positive. What is the correct diagnosis?
    (a) Synovial sarcoma
    (b) Clear cell renal cell carcinoma
    (c) Myoepithelial carcinoma
    (d) Clear cell sarcoma
    (e) Leiomyosarcoma

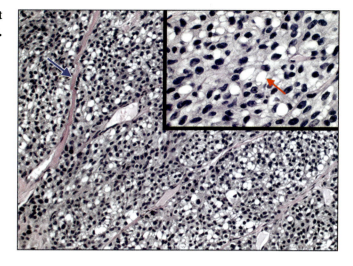

13. A 24-year-old man with a history of cancer involving the left calf presents with a GI bleed and a 3 cm small bowel lesion. What is the correct diagnosis?
    (a) Alveolar rhabdomyosarcoma
    (b) Extraskeletal myxoid chondrosarcoma
    (c) Granular cell tumor
    (d) Alveolar soft part sarcoma
    (e) Metastatic renal cell carcinoma

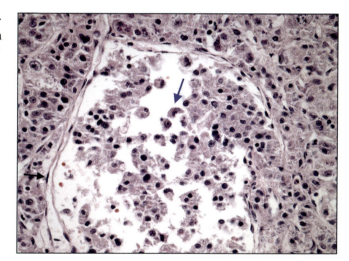

14. A 33-year-old has multiple yellow masses on his right hand along the radial portion of the bilateral second metacarpal phalangeal joints. What is the most specific correct diagnosis?
    (a) Tuberous xanthoma
    (b) Verruciform xanthoma
    (c) Xanthoma
    (d) Granular cell tumor
    (e) Pleomorphic liposarcoma

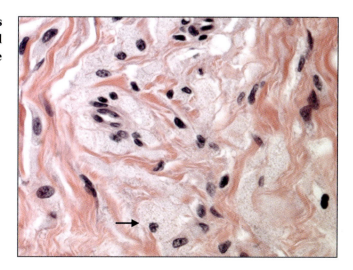

15. **A 28-year-old female has the right thigh lesion depicted here. What does the tumor most likely stain positively for?**
    - (a) MyoD1
    - (b) EMA
    - (c) TFE3
    - (d) Cytokeratin
    - (e) Synaptophysin

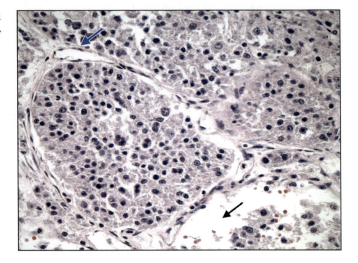

16. **A 71-year-old man with a history of ipsilateral renal cell carcinoma has a slowly growing 1.1 cm left adrenal/peri-adrenal mass. Tumor cells shown to the right are Melan-A positive. What is the correct diagnosis?**
    - (a) Recurrent renal cell carcinoma
    - (b) Dedifferentiated liposarcoma
    - (c) Malignant PEComa
    - (d) Adrenal cortical adenoma
    - (e) Pheochromocytoma

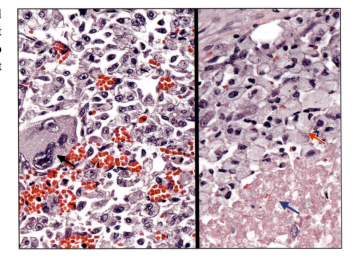

17. **A 19-year-old female with 2 months of abdominal pain presents with a left ovarian mass which is continuous with the small bowel. Tumor cells stain positively for S-100 and HMB-45. What confirmatory test could be ordered next?**
    - (a) C-kit stain
    - (b) Desmin stain
    - (c) Molecular testing for the EWS-ATF1 fusion
    - (d) Molecular testing for SYT-SSX
    - (e) CD99 stain

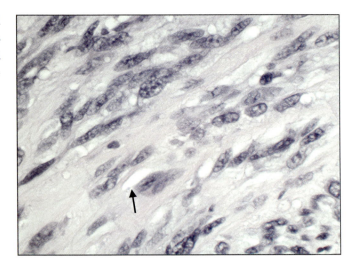

18. **A 4-year-old has a stable non-tender 1 cm left chest wall mass that is depicted to the right. The cells stain positively for S-100. What is the correct diagnosis?**
    (a) Fibroxanthoma
    (b) Fetal rhabdomyoma
    (c) Langerhans cell histiocytosis
    (d) Granular cell tumor
    (e) Hibernoma

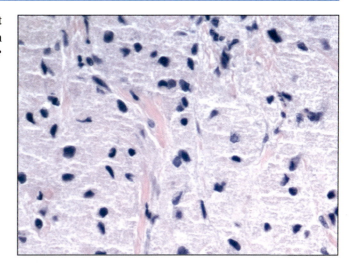

19. **An Ashkenazi Jewish 8-year-old female with a history of lymphoblastic lymphoma that has recurred has a bone marrow biopsy performed. Radiographically, distal femoral metaphyseal widening consistent with an Erlenmeyer flask deformity is seen. What is the correct diagnosis?**
    (a) Recurrent lymphoblastic lymphoma
    (b) Acute myeloid leukemia
    (c) Chronic myeloid leukemia
    (d) Gaucher disease
    (e) Niemann Pick Disease

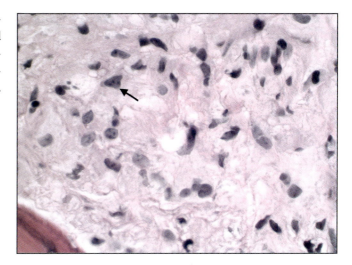

20. **This tumor stains positively for S-100. What type of testing can distinguish between this lesion and malignant melanoma?**
    (a) HMB45 stain
    (b) Melan-A stain
    (c) MiTF stain
    (d) Cytogenetics for t(12;22) translocation
    (e) Cytogenetics for t(11;22) translocation

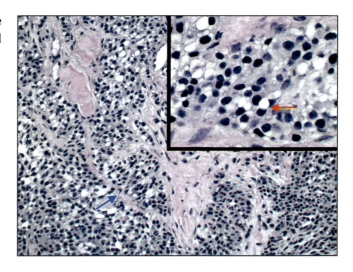

21. A 65-year-old female has bilateral masses at the carotid bifurcation with histology as shown to the right. What stain most likely highlights the cells near the blue arrow?

(a) Synaptophysin

(b) Calcitonin

(c) CD99

(d) AE1/AE3

(e) Thyroglobulin

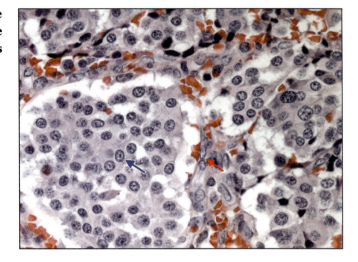

22. A 52-year-old female has had a year of pain near her coccyx. Imaging shows a 4 cm S4-5 lesion restricted to the bone. Histology from the lesion is shown to the right. What is the correct diagnosis?

(a) Chordoma

(b) Pleomorphic liposarcoma

(c) Myxoid liposarcoma

(d) Round cell liposarcoma

(e) Hibernoma

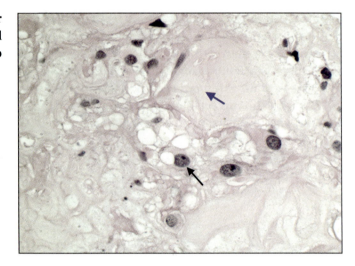

23. A 69-year-old female with a history of neurofibromatosis presents with painful left distal thumb and middle finger lesions. A Melan-A stain is negative. What is the correct diagnosis?

(a) Neurofibroma

(b) Hemangioma

(c) Glomus tumor

(d) PEComa

(e) Glomangioma

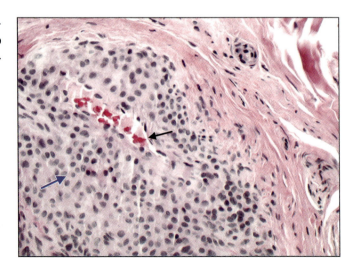

24. What is the most common site for this lesion?

   (a) Skin

   (b) Gastrointestinal tract

   (c) Eyelid

   (d) Genitourinary tract

   (e) Mouth

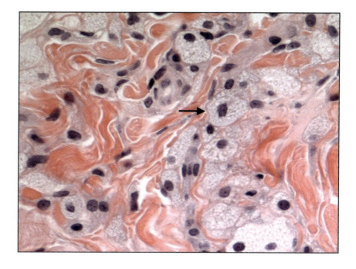

25. A 60-year-old man has a right arm anterior compartment mass. The atypical cell to the right stains positively for desmin and this type of cell is found throughout the tumor. What is the correct diagnosis?

   (a) Pleomorphic undifferentiated sarcoma

   (b) MPNST

   (c) Embryonal rhabdomyosarcoma

   (d) Alveolar rhabdomyosarcoma

   (e) Pleomorphic rhabdomyosarcoma

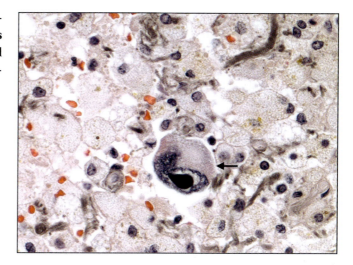

26. A 32-year-old female has a right wrist soft tissue mass containing cells which are Melan-A and HMB45 negative. What is the correct diagnosis?

   (a) Clear cell sarcoma

   (b) Neurothekeoma

   (c) Metastatic renal cell carcinoma

   (d) Metastatic lobular breast carcinoma

   (e) Myoepithelioma

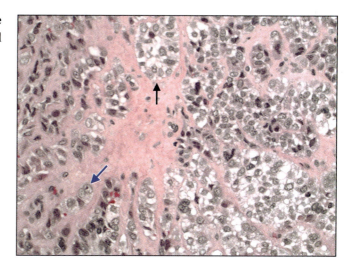

27. **A 36-year-old female has the left buttock lesion depicted here. What translocation is the tumor positive for?**
    (a) T(X;18)
    (b) T(X;17)
    (c) T(11;22)
    (d) T(9;22)
    (e) T(17;22)

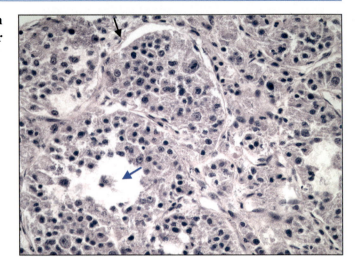

28. **A 74-year-old man has a skull base mass in the left inferotemporal fossa extending to left maxillary sinus and mandibular ramus with bone destruction and muscle involvement. The cells are focally positive for EMA and negative for pancytokeratin, CD34, and HMB-45. What is the correct diagnosis?**
    (a) Sclerosing epithelioid fibrosarcoma
    (b) Hemangiopericytoma
    (c) Metastatic signet ring gastric adenocarcinoma
    (d) Synovial sarcoma
    (e) Clear cell sarcoma

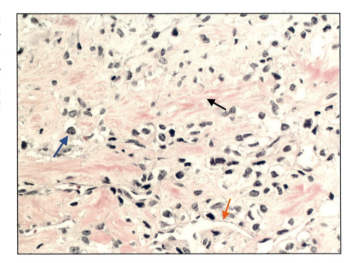

29. **This tumor is encountered most commonly in which region?**
    (a) Arm
    (b) Leg
    (c) Retroperitoneal
    (d) Joint
    (e) Head

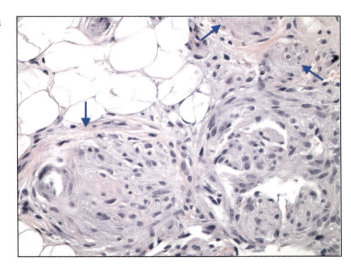

30. **A 2 cm lesion is found in the uterus of a 43-year-old woman. What stain will most likely highlight these cells?**

(a) HMB-45

(b) PAX-8

(c) AE1/AE3

(d) Synaptophysin

(e) GFAP

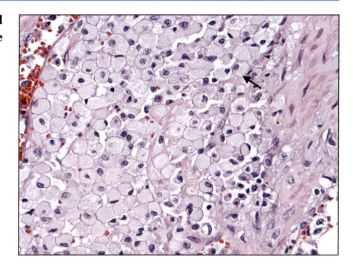

31. **A 50-year-old female has a left middle finger lesion. What is the correct diagnosis?**

(a) Malignant melanoma

(b) Angiosarcoma

(c) Angiomatoid fibrous histiocytoma

(d) Pigmented villonodular synovitis (PVNS)

(e) Langerhans cell histiocytosis

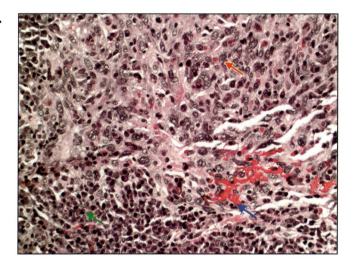

32. **Which cytogenetic events is this lesion associated with?**

(a) Rearrangements of 11q13-21

(b) Loss of 16q, 13q

(c) Amplification of MDM2, CDK4

(d) Ring chromosomes and giant marker chromosomes

(e) Complex multifocal changes

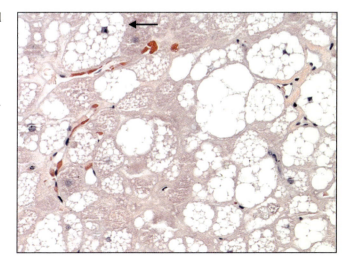

33. A 25-year-old man has a 2 cm right hand soft tissue mass depicted to the right. It is biopsied, diagnosed as granuloma annulare, and the patient is lost to follow-up. Five years later the patient collapses at home and an autopsy shows multiple lung lesions and lymphadenopathy. The original biopsy is reviewed and shown to the right. What stain, if performed at the time of biopsy, could have saved this patient?
    (a) TLE1
    (b) S-100
    (c) HMB-45
    (d) Myogenin
    (e) AE1/AE3

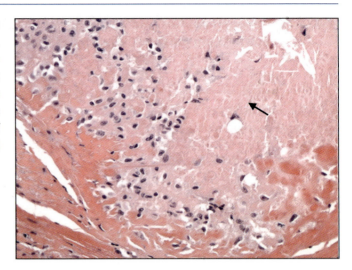

34. A 38-year-old man presented with a right buccal 2 cm nodule. What stain will most likely highlight these cells?
    (a) Muscle specific actin
    (b) S-100
    (c) EMA
    (d) Cytokeratin
    (e) CD68

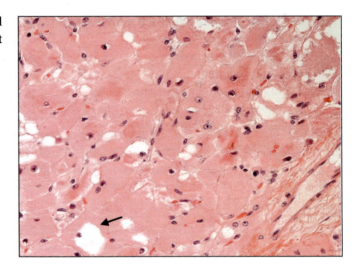

35. A 48-year-old female has a 6.2 cm lesion at the left base of the tongue. An excisional biopsy is done and shown to the right. What is the correct diagnosis?
    (a) Pheochromocytoma
    (b) Paraganglioma
    (c) Squamous cell carcinoma
    (d) Hemangioma
    (e) Salivary canalicular adenoma

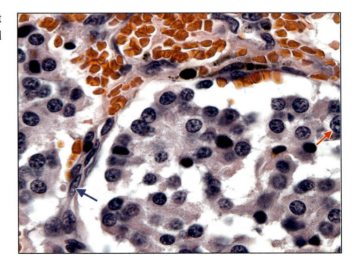

36. Which of the following stains highlights the nodular lesional cells depicted here?

(a) CD68
(b) SMA
(c) Desmin
(d) S-100
(e) Pancytokeratin

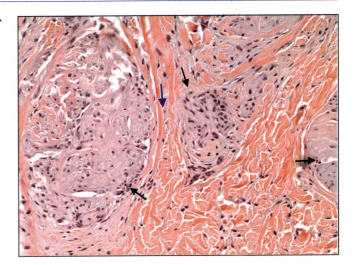

ANSWERS

1. **(c) Juvenile xanthogranuloma**

   The image depicts the main histologic features of juvenile xanthogranuloma including sheets of bland histiocytes, some of which are lipidized (blue arrow) and some of which are not lipidized (red arrow). Giant cells, often of the touton-type, are seen associated with this lesion (black arrow). Myxoid liposarcoma would have a delicate vasculature. Pleomorphic liposarcoma would feature more atypia. Langerhans cell histiocytosis is a close differential but it is often associated with an eosinophilic infiltrate and exhibits cells with longitudinal grooves. Lipidization is not a feature of Langerhans cell histiocytosis. CD117 negativity and the lack of eosinophils and lymphocytes make mastocytosis unlikely.

2. **(a) Malignant extrarenal rhabdoid tumor**

   This is a high power view of a malignant extrarenal rhabdoid tumor. Characteristic features include atypical polygonal cells with voluminous eosinophilic cytoplasm and eccentric nuclei (black arrows) with occasional prominent nucleoli. The eosinophilic cytoplasm contains occasional hyaline inclusions (blue arrow). The ultrastructural findings are consistent with the diagnosis since the hyaline nodules display intermediate fibers with a vague whorling pattern by electron microscopy. This tumor occurs most often in infants and children. Oncocytoma has nuclei that are more central and regular. Granular cell tumor would display more granularity to the cytoplasm. Chromophobe renal cell carcinoma occurs in the elderly and would not display these ultrastructural features. Multiple myeloma would show eccentric nuclei without the eosinophilic hue and is not consistent with the ultrastructural findings.

3. **(a) Adult rhabdomyoma**

   Adult rhabdomyoma is characterized by regular polygonal cells with abundant eosinophilic cytoplasm and occasionally vacuolated cytoplasm (black arrow). The head and neck is the most common site for this tumor and it affects adults. Granular cell tumor can also be found in the esophagus but would have more granular cytoplasm. Hibernoma would most likely feature polyvacuolated cells and the upper back is the most common site. Fetal rhabdomyoma features muscle fibers with a variable amount of myxoid background, not polygonal cells. Pleomorphic rhabdomyosarcoma would show marked cellular atypia not seen here.

4. **(e) Loss of INI1**

   This is a malignant extrarenal rhabdoid tumor because numerous rhabdoid cells are present with polygonal contours, abundant eosinophilic cytoplasm, and eccentric nuclei. Characteristic intracytoplasmic eosinophilic inclusions are also seen (black arrow). Most malignant extrarenal rhabdoid tumors feature loss of INI1. They do not show S100 staining but stain positively for pancytokeratin, vimentin, and EMA,

5. **(a) EMA**

   The image displays epithelioid cells many of which have an intracytoplasmic lumen and some of the intracytoplasmic lumens contain red blood cells (red arrow). The tumor cells are embedded in a hyalinized or occasionally myxoid stroma. These histologic findings and the radiographic history of multiple lesions affecting the same bone favors epithelioid hemangioendothelioma. This tumor displays staining for the more specific markers, Fli-1, CD31, and CD34. Also, nearly half of these tumors display CK7 staining, leading to diagnostic confusion with a carcinoma. Epithelioid hemangioendothelioma rarely expresses EMA.

6. **(b) Xanthoma**

   Xanthoma shows aggregates of foamy histiocytes (black arrow) as seen in the image. Verruciform xanthoma demonstrates parakeratosis and papillary structures which are not seen here. Tuberous xanthoma occurs at tendinous sites. The remaining choices do not feature foamy histiocytes.

7. **(c) Hibernoma**

   This is a hibernoma with regions of mature white fat admixed with brightly eosinophilic mitochondria-filled brown fat cells (black arrow) and polyvesiculated brown fat cells (blue arrow). Lipoma and spindle cell lipoma do not display cells with eosinophilic cytoplasm or polyvesiculated cells. Atypical lipoma cells would display more nuclear atypia. Granular cell tumor features cells with granular, eosinophilic cytoplasm. There is no granularity to this homogenous eosinophilic cytoplasm.

8. **(a) T(2;22)**

    This lesion is angiomatoid fibrous histiocytoma. The image shows a nodule of histiocytoid cells (red arrow) circumferentially lined by a rim of chronic inflammation (green arrow), which is typical for this lesion. Among the histiocytoid cells, characteristic microhemorrhages can be seen (blue arrow). Desmin is positive in approximately half of these cases. The tranlocation t(2;22) of EWSR1-CREB1 is seen in over half of angiomatoid fibrous histiocytomas. T(12;22) and t(12;16) are less frequent tranlocations. T(11;22) is seen in desmoplastic small round blue cell tumor and t(X;17) is found in alveolar soft part sarcoma.

9. **(c) Calcifying fibrous tumor**

    This lesion is composed of a fibrous stroma with epithelioid fibroblasts (green arrow), abundant chronic inflammatory cells (blue arrow), and occasional calcifications (black arrow), all of which are characteristic features of calcifying fibrous tumor. Desmoplastic fibroblastoma also has a paucicellular fibroblastic network; however, it lacks calcifications. Leiomyoma with degenerative changes could exhitibt calcifications but would stain for desmin. Metastatic lobular breast carcinoma in a patient this young would be rare. Plexiform fibromyxoma is found in the stomach and would not feature calcifications.

10. **(b) Plexiform fibrohistiocytic tumor**

    Plexiform fibrohistiocytic tumor has nodules of epithelioid and histiocytic cells (black arrows), exhibiting large amounts of amphophilic cytoplasm. The intervening collagenous tissue (red arrow) contains bland fibroblasts. Tuberculosis and epithelioid sarcoma would contain nodules with central necrosis. Granuloma annulare would feature central necrobiotic collagen. Sarcoidosis would not feature the interspersed bland fibroblastic proliferation seen in this image.

11. **(c) Epithelioid sarcoma**

    Epithelioid sarcoma shows a nodular growth pattern of cells with eosinophilic cytoplasm surrounding centrally necrotic zones (black arrow), giving it a granulomatous appearance. Thus, granuloma annulare and necrobiosis lipoidica are often in the differential diagnosis, both of which contain necrotic regions bordered by palisading histiocytes. It is prudent to get a cytokeratin stain when confronted with a centrally necrotic epithelioid lesion especially near the hand (the most common site of epithelioid sarcoma) as negativity will easily rule out epithelioid sarcoma. Loss of INI1 is found in most epithelioid sarcomas but is not specific for epithelioid sarcoma. A cytokeratin stain will not highlight military tuberculosis, granuloma annulare, or necrobiosis lipoidica. An infarction would not contain epithelioid cells surrounding necrotic regions.

12. **(d) Clear cell sarcoma**

    Clear cell sarcoma contains nests and sheets of cells with glycogenated cytoplasm (red arrow) separated by thin fibrous strands (blue arrow). This tumor typically occurs in patients in their second or third decade and the lower extremity is the most likely site. The other tumors listed do not stain for HMB45 and Melan-A.

13. **(d) Alveolar soft part sarcoma**

    As seen in the image, alveolar soft part sarcoma features nests of polygonal cells with eosinophilic cytoplasm which are occasionally discohesive (blue arrow). The nests are separated by thin vascular spaces with a unicellular lining (black arrow). This tumor typically first occurs in the lower extremities of young adult patients, as in this example. Alveolar rhabdomyosarcoma would have a pseudo-alveolar growth pattern with thick fibrous septae between nests instead of a unicellular layer. Additionally, alveolar rhabdomyosarcoma is a small round blue cell tumor and would not feature the abundant eosinophilic cytoplasm seen here. Eosinophilic cells would be present in extraskeletal myxoid chondrosarcoma; however, these would be cords and nests of eosinophilic cells deposited in a myxoid matrix which is not seen here. A granular cell tumor would not show this nesting pattern or dyscohesion. Metastatic renal cell carcinoma is a close differential since it also can have a nested pattern with eosinophilic cells; however, the dyscohesion and clinical history in this case is not consistent with metastatic renal cell carcinoma.

14. **(a) Tuberous xanthoma**

Tuberous xanthoma is a tendon-associated xanthoma frequently found on the buttocks, elbow joint, knee joint, ankle joint, or over carpal, metacarpal, or interphalangeal joints in the hand. The image depicts lipid-laden histiocytes (black arrow), consistent with xanthoma. This is not a verruciform xanthoma because there are no papillary structures or hyperkeratosis. Granular cell tumor is unlikely because the cells are not granular or eosinophilic. Xanthoma is technically correct, but the location of the lesion, over a hand joint, allows us to use the more specific designation, tuberous xanthoma. Pleomorphic liposarcoma would show more atpia.

15. **(c) TFE3**

This is an alveolar soft part sarcoma. The clinical history of a young patient with a lower extremity tumor points to the diagnosis. The image shows the characteristic unicellular vascular spaces (blue arrow) separating nests of discohesive polygonal tumor cells with abundant amphophilic cytoplasm. The dyscohesion can lead to a pseudo-alveolar appearance (black arrow). Alveolar soft part sarcomas stain negatively for all the markers listed except TFE3.

16. **(c) Malignant PEComa**

This PEComa shows characteristic sheets of ovoid Melan-A positive cells with abundant clear to eosinophilic cytoplasm (red arrow). Occasional cells with markedly atypical nuclei (black arrow) are seen as well as necrosis (blue arrow), making this a malignant PEComa. Recurrent renal cell carcinoma would likely show more of a nested pattern. Dedifferentiated liposarcoma would show a well-differentiated liposarcoma component. Adrenal cortical adenoma would not likely show necrosis or this degree of atypia. Pheochromocytoma would have more of a nested architecture. All of the answer choices besides malignant PEComa are Melan-A negative

17. **(c) Molecular testing for the EWS-ATF1 fusion**

This is morphologically and immunophenotypically consistent with clear cell sarcoma. Clear cell sarcoma can have epithelioid or spindled tumor cells with prominent cytoplasmic glycogenation (black arrow). As in this case, they stain for melanocytic markers. This is not a typical site for clear cell sarcoma (deep extremity soft tissue is the preferred site) so if there was still uncertainty after the immunohistologic workup a molecular test for the EWS-ATF1 translocation can be ordered which is present in the vast majority of clear cell sarcomas. C-kit staining would help to diagnose a GIST which would not be expected to stain positively for S-100. Desmin would highlight leiomyosarcoma or leiomyoma which would not show S-100 staining or glycogenated cytoplasm. SYT-SSX and CD99 testing would help to diagnose a synovial sarcoma which would not be expected to stain for S-100.

18. **(d) Granular cell tumor**

Granular cell tumor, composed of polygonal cells with abundant granular amphophilic cytoplasm, typically occurs in the tongue and superficial soft tissues of the upper body. Granular cell tumors stain positively for S-100. Fetal rhabdomyoma would have spindled cells and striations. Langerhans cell histiocytosis would show a prominent inflammatory infiltrate with scattered grooved langerhans cells. Hibernoma would feature polyvesiculated or eosinophilic brown fat with at least some amount of intermixed white fat.

19. **(d) Gaucher disease**

Radiographically, the presence of a Erlenmeyer flask deformity is typical of Gaucher disease. Histologically, the diagnostic findings of a proliferation of histiocytoid cells with small eccentric nuclei surrounded by abundant pink cytoplasm (Gaucher cells, black arrow) replacing the marrow are seen. Leukemias and lymphomas would show infiltration by cells that are not histiocytoid. Niemann Pick Disease shows infiltration by foam cells, not Gaucher cells.

20. **(d) Cytogenetics for t(12;22) translocation**

This is a clear cell sarcoma from the histologic findings of glycogenated cells (red arrow) and fibrous strands (blue arrow) separating nests and sheets of cells. Clear cell sarcoma stains positively for melanocytic markers, creating diagnostic confusion with metastatic melanoma. The histology in this case favors clear cell sarcoma but in less clear cut cases, due to the fact that both lesions stain positively for S-100, HMB45, Melan-A, and MiTF, cytogenetics for the t(12;22) translocation should be performed. This translocation of the *EWS* gene into ATF1 is not found in melanoma.

21. **(a) Synaptophysin**

The carotid bifurcation is a common location for paraganglioma which contains nests of cells with stippled chromatin (blue arrow) encircled by spindled sustentacular cells (red arrow). Paragangliomas stain positively for synaptophysin, chromogranin, and CD56. The remaining answer choices do not stain paraganglioma.

22. (a) Chordoma

Chordoma arises from central bony sites with preference for the skull or sacrum. Histologically, bubbly vacuolated physaliferous cells are seen (black arrow) deposited in an edematous myxoid stroma (blue arrow). Pleomorphic liposarcoma would have more atypia. Myxoid liposarcoma would have a more vascular component. Round cell liposarcoma would be more cellular and not have physaliferous cells. Hibernoma would have polyvacuolated cells but the vacuoles would be smaller and there would be some associated white fat.

23. (c) Glomus tumor

The image depicts a glomus tumor with regular round cells with abundant amphophilic cytoplasm (blue arrow) evenly distributed around a vascular channel (black arrow). The most common site for a glomus tumor is the finger. The cellular component is much more significant than the vascular component, ruling out glomangioma and hemangioma. PEComa would show Melan-A positivity. Neurofibroma would show cells with wavy nuclei and the tumor cells would not be perivascular.

24. (a) Skin

This is a xanthoma, recognizable by the aggregates of foamy histiocytes (black arrow). Xanthomas are most often found on the skin. They can be associated with tendons, in which case they are named tuberous xanthomas. They can also be associated with the eyelid. The gastrointestinal tract, genitourinary tract, and mouth are less likely sites for xanthomas.

25. (e) Pleomorphic rhabdomyosarcoma

This is most likely a pleomorphic rhabdomyosarcoma. The large atypical cell in the center (black arrow) is a markedly atypical rhabdomyoblast with eosinophilic cytoplasm, an eccentric nucleus, and a prominent enlarged nucleolus. It is much larger than most of its neighboring cells and is consistent with pleomorphic rhabdomyosarcoma. The staining pattern is also consistent with pleomorphic rhabdomyosarcoma, with the vast majority staining positively for desmin. These tumors typically occur in adults as in this case. Pleomorphic undifferentiated sarcoma would not show desmin positivity. MPNST would not show rhabdomyoblastic features. Embryonal rhabdomyosarcoma can exhibit rhabdomyoblasts; however, there should be some histologic signs of embryonal rhabdomyosarcoma such as alternating hypercellular and hypocellular areas. The architecture of alveolar rhabdomyosarcoma is not present.

26. (e) Myoepithelioma

Myoepithelioma can have a variety of apperances. The lesion typically consists of epithelial cells deposited in nests (black arrow) and cords (blue arrow) with some cells displaying a physaliferous cytoplasm (black arrow). Clear cell sarcoma, also known as melanoma of soft parts, would likely be positive for HMB45 and may show Melan-A positivity. Neurothekeoma and renal cell carcinoma would not form cords. Metastatic lobular breast cancer would not have such a physaliferous appearance.

27. (b) T(X;17)

This is a alveolar soft part sarcoma. Diagnostic features include nested cells with abundant eosinophilic cytoplasm and dyscohesion (blue arrow). Nests are separated by unicellularly-lined vascular spaces (black arrow). Alveolar soft part sarcoma is associated with T(X;17) that translocates the *TFE3* gene to the ASPL locus, producing an abnormal transcription factor. T(X;18) is found in synovial sarcoma. T(11;22) is found in Ewing's sarcoma. T(9;22) is found in chronic myeloid leukemia. T(17;22) is found in dermatofibrosarcoma protuberans.

28. (a) Sclerosing epithelioid fibrosarcoma

Sclerosing epithelioid fibrosarcoma is characterized by epithelioid nests, chords, and single cells with a clear/vacuolated (blue arrow) to eosinophilic cytoplasm which are haphazardly embedded in a dense eosinophilic collagenous matrix (black arrow). Irregularly shaped hemangiopericytoma-type vessels can occasionally be seen in this lesion (red arrow). These tumors are occasionally positive for EMA but are negative for most other markers. Pancytokeratin negativity rules out gastric adenocarcinoma. Hemangiopericytoma would be CD34 positive. Synovial sarcoma would be more spindled and hypercellular than this. Clear cell sarcoma is a close differential due to the presence of clear cells; however, the density of collagen and HMB-45 negativity makes clear cell sarcoma unlikely.

29. (a) Arm

This lesion is a plexiform fibrohistiocytic tumor, with a minimal fibrous stromal component. The critical feature of multiple epithelioid-histiocytic cell nodules (blue arrows) is present with no central necrosis or surrounding inflammation that would trigger a different differential diagnosis. These nodules can sometimes extend into the subcutaneous tissue, as is seen in this case. The most likely place for these tumors to arise is the arm, followed by the leg.

30. **(a) HMB-45**

This is a PEComa. Diagnostic histologic findings include clusters of ovoid cells (black arrow) with light pink eosinophilic cytoplasm. PEComas are known to stain both for melanocytic markers and smooth muscle markers. HMB-45 is positive in the vast majority of cases. The other listed stains are negative in PEComa.

31. **(c) Angiomatoid fibrous histiocytoma**

Angiomatoid fibrous histiocytoma is a lesion composed of histiocytoid nodules (red arrow) admixed with microhemorrhages (blue arrow), hemosiderin deposition, and circumferentially lined by a dense inflammatory infiltrate (green arrow). Malignant melanoma would not feature histiocytoid cells. The nuclear features of the histiocytoid cells are too regular for angiosarcoma. Pigmented villonodular synovitis features hemosiderin deposition and histiocytoid cells; however, PVNS should have abundant giant cells and hemosiderin deposition. Langerhans cell histiocytosis would show more of an eosinophilic infiltrate.

32. **(a) Rearrangements of 11q13-21**

This is a hibernoma. The large polyvesiculated cells with central nuclei (black arrow) represent the brown fat component of a hibernoma. Hibernomas are associated with rearrangements of chromosomal region 11q13-21. Loss of 16q, 13q is seen in spindle cell lipoma but this case shows no spindle cell population. Ring chromosomes, giant marker chromosomes, and amplification of MDM2 and CDK4 are present in well-differentiated liposarcoma that would show more atypia. Complex multifocal changes are seen in pleomorphic liposarcoma that would show more atypia. None of the lesions except hibernoma shows brown fat.

33. **(e) AE1/AE3**

Epithelioid sarcoma most often involves the hands of young patients. Histologically, it demonstrates nodules of cells with eosinophilic cytoplasm surrounding necrotic regions (black arrow). A close benign histologic mimic is granuloma annulare which shows palisaded histiocytes surrounding central necrobiotic collagen. Immunohistochemistry for AE1/AE3 and CD68 should have been performed as granuloma annulare will not stain for AE1/AE3 and epithelioid sarcoma will not stain for CD68. Atypical for sarcomas, epithelioid sarcoma shows both lymphatic and hematogenous spread.

34. **(a) Muscle specific actin**

This is an adult rhabdomyoma. Histologic features shown include polygonal deeply eosinophilic cells with occasional vacuolations (black arrow). The oral cavity is a typical site for this tumor. Nearly all adult rhabdomyomas stain positively for myoglobin and muscle specific actin. These lesions can occasionally stain for S-100. They are negative for EMA, cytokeratin, and CD68.

35. **(b) Paraganglioma**

This is a paraganglioma with nests of cells with finely stippled chromatin (red arrow) and spindled circumscribing sustentacular cells (blue arrow). These nests give the tumor a "Zellballen" appearance, appearing to be multiple small balls. Pheochromocytoma outside of the adrenal gland is called paraganglioma. Squamous cell carcinoma can have a nested appearance but would not feature stippled chromatin and sustentacular cells. Hemangioma would show defined vascular spaces as the main component of the lesion. Canalicular adenoma would have a trabecular architecture with more basaloid cells.

36. **(a) CD68**

This is a plexiform fibrohistiocytic tumor with epithelioid to histiocytic nodules of cells with abundant amphophilic cytoplasm (black arrow) and intervening bland fibroblasts (blue arrow). CD68 highlights the nodular cells in plexiform fibrohistiocytic tumor. SMA can show positivity in the fibrous component but is negative in the nodules. Pancytokeratin would be positive in an epithelioid sarcoma but there is no necrosis that would suggest that diagnosis. Desmin and S-100 are negative in this tumor.

CHAPTER 7

Lytic and Cystic Lesions of Bones and Joints

1. **A 39-year-old female has a cortical lesion in the proximal tibia. The pre-biopsy differential diagnosis includes ossifying fibroma, metastasis, and nonossifying fibroma. What is the correct diagnosis?**
   - (a) Ossifying fibroma
   - (b) Metastatic carcinoma
   - (c) Nonossifying fibroma
   - (d) Osteofibrous dysplasia
   - (e) Fibrous dysplasia

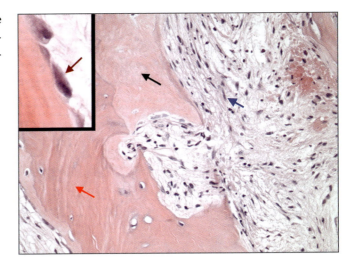

2. **A 36-year-old female has a left knee cyst that communicates with the synovial space. Histology from the excision specimen is shown to the right. All of the following diagnoses have been used to describe lesions with similar pathophysiology in the knee and elsewhere in the body except?**
   - (a) Baker's cyst
   - (b) Ganglion cyst
   - (c) Popliteal cyst
   - (d) Synovial cyst
   - (e) Spinal cyst

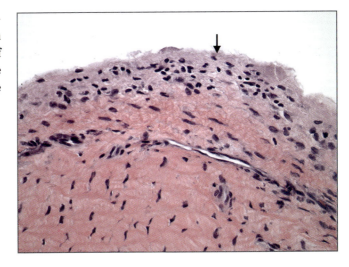

3. **A 3-year-old girl has a 2 cm lytic lesion in the left lateral C1 vertebral body laterally displacing the carotid and vertebral arteries. The radiologic differential diagnosis is rhabdomyosarcoma vs leukemia. What is the correct diagnosis?**
   - (a) Alveolar rhabdomyosarcoma
   - (b) Chronic osteomyelitis
   - (c) Acute osteomyelitis
   - (d) Langerhans cell histiocytosis
   - (e) Disseminated Hodgkin's disease

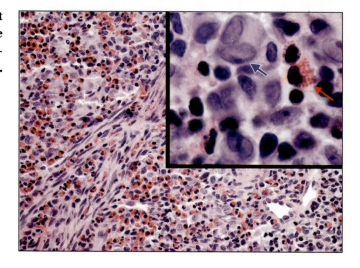

4. **A 31-year-old female has a mass on the dorsum of her right wrist. A cyst is removed which has the lining shown. Which of the following is the main risk factor for this disease process?**
   - (a) Radiation
   - (b) Chemotherapy
   - (c) Trauma
   - (d) Degenerative joint disease
   - (e) Lymphedema

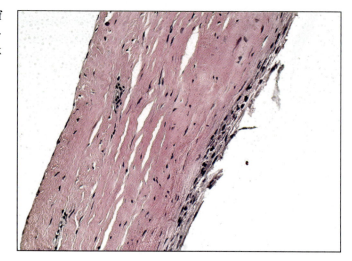

5. **A 9-year-old boy displays an expansile radiolucent lesion in the distal fibular metadiaphysis with some periosteal reaction and bony remodeling associated with a pathologic fracture after fall. The lesion is depicted to the right. What is the correct diagnosis?**
   - (a) Nonossifying fibroma
   - (b) Fibrous dysplasia
   - (c) Telangiectatic osteosarcoma
   - (d) Giant cell tumor of bone
   - (e) Aneurysmal bone cyst

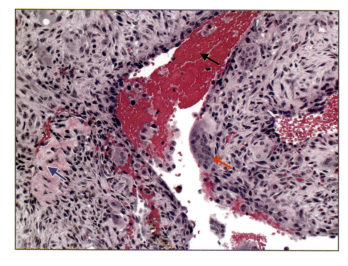

6. **A 38-year-old woman has a painful 9 mm inferior iliac spine lytic, cystic lesion with no involvement of neighboring soft tissue shown to the right. The lesion is hyperintense and enhances. Lab tests show a markedly elevated PTH. What is the most likely diagnosis?**
   - (a) Aneurysmal bone cyst
   - (b) Giant cell tumor of bone
   - (c) Brown tumor
   - (d) Nonossifying fibroma
   - (e) Undifferentiated pleomorphic sarcoma with giant cells

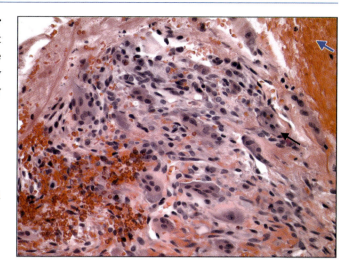

7. **A 40-year-old female has a nonaggressive-appearing sclerotic lesion at the anterior-lateral portion of the proximal tibial diaphysis. There is a slight periosteal elevation adjacent to the lesion with no soft tissue mass identified. The radiologist feels this could represent osteofibrous dysplasia. What is the correct diagnosis?**
   - (a) Adamantinoma
   - (b) Fibrous dysplasia
   - (c) Osteofibrous dysplasia
   - (d) Ossifying fibroma
   - (e) Nonossifying fibroma

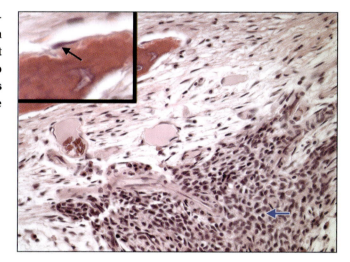

8. **A 50-year-old man found a 1.3 cm bump in the left frontal bone that was radiographically stable for some time until the patient opted to have it removed. On high power increased osteoclastic activity is seen. Histology from the lesion is shown to the right. What is the correct diagnosis?**
   - (a) Benign bone
   - (b) Bone island
   - (c) Fibrous dysplasia
   - (d) Paget's disease of bone
   - (e) Brown tumor

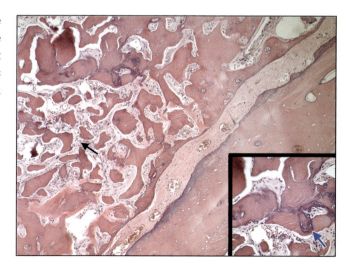

9. **A 14-year-old female has right leg pain and imaging shows a distal tibial lytic metaphyseal lesion with a rim that is sclerotic. The histology for this well-circumscribed lesion is shown to the right. What is the correct diagnosis?**
   - (a) Giant cell tumor of bone
   - (b) Desmoplastic fibroma
   - (c) Fibrous dysplasia
   - (d) Aneurysmal bone cyst
   - (e) Nonossifying fibroma

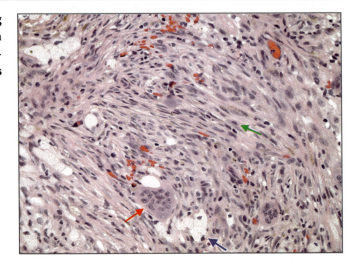

10. **An 11-year-old boy has a right humeral medullary metaphysis unilocular cystic lesion on radiology with the histologic appearance shown to the right. What is the correct diagnosis?**
    - (a) Intraosseous ganglion cyst
    - (b) Subchondral cyst
    - (c) Unicameral bone cyst
    - (d) Aneurysmal bone cyst
    - (e) Fracture callus

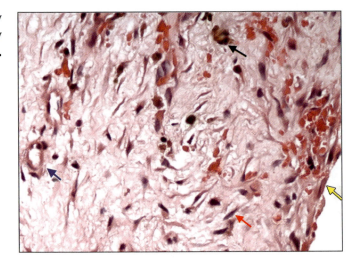

11. **A 50-year-old female has a cyst above the left wrist. Surgically, the cyst does not communicate with the joint cavity. What is the correct diagnosis?**
    - (a) Baker's cyst
    - (b) Ganglion cyst (extraosseous)
    - (c) Juxta-articular myxoma
    - (d) Cysticercosis
    - (e) Subchondral cyst

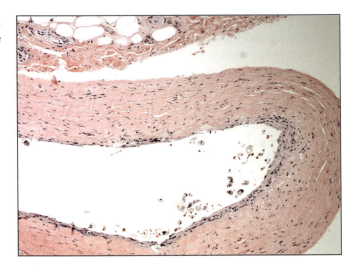

12. A 57-year-old female had a fall from standing and fractured her right humeral shaft. Imaging studies showed an isolated lytic lesion. The excision specimen is shown to the right and a CD138 stain is shown in the inset. What is the correct diagnosis?
    (a) Plasma cell neoplasm
    (b) Metastatic PEComa
    (c) Metastatic melanoma
    (d) Pleomorphic undifferentiated sarcoma
    (e) Osteoblastic osteosarcoma

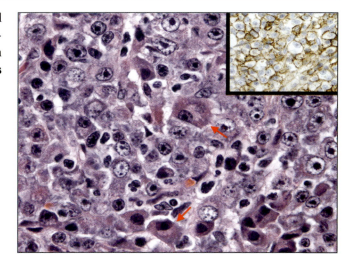

13. A 13-year-old male has had right knee pain for six months that is present with motion and at rest. Imaging shows a proximal tibial epiphyseal lytic lesion. There is a sclerotic rim around the lesion. What is the correct diagnosis?
    (a) Chondroblastoma
    (b) Nonossifying fibroma
    (c) Giant cell tumor of bone
    (d) Aneurysmal bone cyst
    (e) Chondromyxoid fibroma

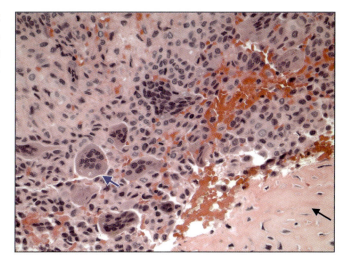

14. A 9-year-old female has been diagnosed with precocious puberty and has multiple lytic left and right tibial medullary lesions shown to the right. What syndrome does she most likely suffer from?
    (a) Down's syndrome
    (b) Carney complex
    (c) McCune-Albright syndrome
    (d) Velocardiofacial syndrome
    (e) Maffucci syndrome

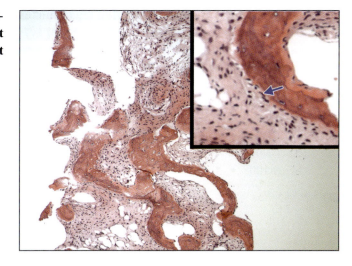

15. **A 30-year-old female has a distal femoral medullary metaphysis lesion depicted to the right. Cytogenetic testing would most likely show?**
    (a) T(11;22)
    (b) Translocation involving 17p13.2
    (c) No changes
    (d) T(X;18)
    (e) Complex cytogenetic changes

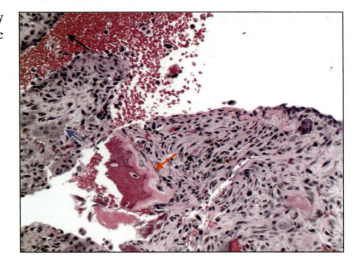

16. **A 33-year-old male, status post ACL reconstruction, now presents with knee stiffness. An MRI shows a joint effusion containing floating leaf-like projections shown to the right. What is the correct diagnosis?**
    (a) Angiolipoma
    (b) Spindle cell lipoma
    (c) Synovial lipomatosis
    (d) Angiomyolipoma
    (e) Hemangioma

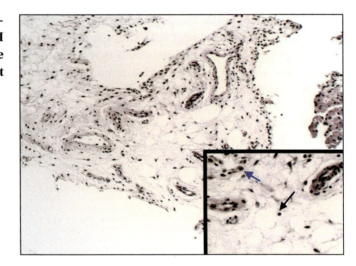

17. **A 10-year-old boy has a scapular mass that is extending into the supraspinatus fossa. A biopsy is shown to the right and ultrastructural studies reveal Birbeck granules. What stain was most likely run in the inset?**
    (a) Cytokeratin
    (b) CD30
    (c) CD15
    (d) HMB45
    (e) S-100

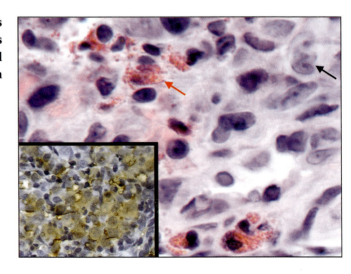

18. **A 51-year-old man with hemophilia has what appears to be a loose body in the knee and undergoes loose body removal. What is the correct diagnosis?**

(a) PVNS
(b) Intrasynovial hemangioma
(c) Hemosiderotic synovitis
(d) Loose body
(e) Malignant melanoma

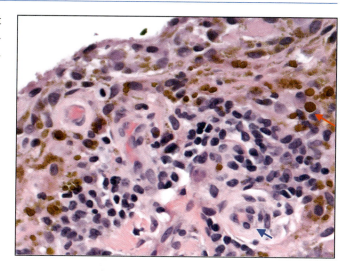

ANSWERS

1. **(d) Osteofibrous dysplasia**
   Osteofibrous dysplasia typically occurs in children younger than the age of 15; thus, the age of this patient is atypical but not unprecedented. The most likely site for osteofibrous dysplasia is a cortical location on the tibia. Histologically, osteofibrous dysplasia features bland spindled cells (blue arrow) associated with immature (black arrow) and more mature bone (red arrow). Prominent osteoblastic rimming can be seen in osteofibrous dysplasia (brown arrow). Ossifying fibroma is typically found in the jaw. There are no groups of cytologically malignant cells, ruling out metastatic carcinoma. Non-ossifying fibroma would not show bone with various levels of maturation and would show giant cells. Fibrous dysplasia is typically medullary, not cortical, and would not show osteoblastic rimming.

2. **(b) Ganglion cyst**
   This case describes a synovial cyst which is a cyst caused by synovial membrane herniation. Keys to the diagnosis include the presence of a synovial lining (black arrow) and the clinical history that the cyst communicates with the synovial space. When this type of cyst is present in the knee it is called a popliteal or Baker's cyst. When present in the spine this cyst is named spinal cyst. Ganglion cysts are mucoid cysts that form either due to degeneration of the joint capsule or overproduction of mucin by fibroblasts, not synovial membrane herniation.

3. **(d) Langerhans cell histiocytosis**
   This lesion is Langerhans cell histiocytosis based on the eosinophilic infiltrate (red arrow) and the binucleated cells with grooves (Langerhans cells, blue arrow). The image shows some fibrous septation; however, alveolar rhabdomyosarcoma is a small round blue cell tumor and should not show Langerhans cells with abundant eosinophilic infiltration. Acute and chronic osteomyelitis should feature neutrophils and plasma cells, respectively; however, the main infiltrate in this case is eosinophils. Disseminated Hodgkin's disease could show an eosinophilic infiltrate with binucleation but Hodgkin's cells would have more prominent nucleoli and Hodgkin's lymphoma would be rare at this age.

4. **(c) Trauma**
   This is a ganglion cyst from the clinical description, a cyst involving the small joints and tendons of the hand, and the histologic image is consistent, depicting a thick fibrous capsule with a thin inner lining. Over half of ganglion cysts are thought to follow a history of trauma. Radiation and lymphedema are risk factors for angiosarcoma. Degenerative joint disease is a risk factor for subchondral cyst which would have granulation tissue or degenerative bone changes associated with it.

5. **(e) Aneurysmal bone cyst**
   This lesion displays blood filled spaces (black arrow) surrounded by spindled fibroblasts intermixed with giant cells (red arrow) and osteoid (blue arrow) which are all features of aneurysmal bone cyst. Importantly, there is no hyperchromasia or overt atypia that would lead to the diagnosis of telangiectatic osteosarcoma. Fibrous dysplasia would not have so many giant cells or blood filled spaces. Giant cell tumor of bone and nonossifying fibroma would not feature large blood filled spaces.

6. **(c) Brown tumor**
   Given the clinical history of hyperparathyroidism, suspicion for brown tumor must be high. Histologic evidence of brown tumor is present including multinucleated giant cells (black arrow) and hemorrhage (blue arrow). The hemorrhage and subsequent hemosiderin deposition gives this tumor its brown appearance and its name. Aneurysmal bone cyst, giant cell tumor of bone, and ossifying fibroma can all have a proliferation of giant cells leading to diagnostic confusion; however, none of the other choices is associated with elevated PTH. There is insufficient cytologic atypia for undifferentiated pleomorphic sarcoma with giant cells.

7. **(a) Adamantinoma**
   This lesion displays irregularly shaped clusters of cytokeratin-positive epithelial cells (blue arrow) deposited in a background of bland spindled cells interspersed with osteoblast-rimmed (black arrow) bony trabeculae, all of

which are features of adamantinoma. Additionally, the tibia is a common site for this tumor. The bland spindled cells and osteoblastic rimming (black arrow) suggest the diagnosis of osteofibrous dysplasia; however, epithelial islands are not a feature of osteofibrous dysplasia. Nevertheless, the distinction between osteofibrous dysplasia (Campanacci's disease) and adamantinoma remains contentious with some believing osteofibrous dysplasia is an adamantinoma which has not been sampled adequately enough to find epithelial islands due to their overlapping clinical presentation and histologic features. Fibrous dysplasia and ossifying fibroma would not feature epithelial nests. Nonossifying fibroma should not have osteoblast-lined bony trabeculae or epithelial nests.

8. (d) Paget's disease of bone

The histology shows an irregular pattern of bone deposition (black arrow) which contains regions of irregular cementum (blue arrow), both diagnostic features of Paget's disease. Benign bone and bone island would not show these features. The irregular bone deposition has an appearance similar to fibrous dysplasia; however, no bland spindled cell population is identified expanding the intertrabecular space and irregular cementum lines is not characteristic for fibrous dysplasia. Brown tumor would show hemorrhage which is not seen.

9. (e) Nonossifying fibroma

This is a nonossifying fibroma. This tumor often occurs in teenage patients as in this questions stem and the metaphysis of a long bone is the most common location. The radiologic findings of a lytic lesion with a sclerotic rim are classic for this lesion. Histologically it is composed of fascicles of bland spindled cells (green arrow) with scattered hemosiderin laden macrophages, clusters of foam cells (blue arrow), and multinucleated giant cells (red arrow). Due to the giant cells, giant cell tumor of bone can arise in the differential; however giant cell tumor of bone would have more giant cells and epiphyseal involvement. Desmoplastic fibroma would not have giant cells or foam cells and radiologically would show a more infiltrative pattern than seen here. Fibrous dysplasia displays curvilinear bony trabeculae and has a predilection for the medulla of bones, not the metaphysis. Giant cells and foam cells can be present in aneurysmal bone cyst; however, aneurysmal bone cyst should show dilated blood filled spaces and new bone formation which is not seen here.

10. (c) Unicameral bone cyst

Unicameral bone cysts typically occur in patients younger than 20 and are found most commonly in the medulla of the metaphysis of the femur or humerus. The cyst lining is atypical, being composed of just a fibrous band in many cases (yellow arrow). Under the fibrous tissue, granulation tissue-type vessels (blue arrow), spindled cells (red arrow), and hemosiderin laden macrophages (black arrow) can be seen in this and many cases of unicameral bone cyst. Intraosseous ganglion cyst would show a myxoid background which is not seen here. Subchondral cyst occurs in the setting of osteoarthritis so the clinical history does not match that diagnosis. Aneurysmal bone cyst typically would show reactive bone, osteoid, and multinucleated giant cells which are not seen. Fracture callus would show fibroblasts with woven bone.

11. (b) Ganglion cyst (extraosseous)

Ganglion cysts are the most common soft tissue lesions of the wrists but can affect other joints as well. Histologically, they feature a thick fibrous capsule with a very thin cyst lining. Baker's cyst would communicate with the joint space. Juxta-articular myxoma occurs in larger joints like the elbow, knee, and hip. Cysticercosis, an infection caused by taenia solium, could feature a cyst with a thick lining; however, inside the cyst suckers and hooklets would be seen. Subchondral cyst would be surrounded by degenerative bone or granulation tissue.

12. (a) Plasma cell neoplasm

Despite the large number of pleomorphic cells some of which have prominent nucleoli, the presence of nearly pancellular membrane CD138 positivity and focally a few more well-differentiated plasma cells with eccentric nuclei and perinuclear clearing (red arrows) makes this a plasma cell neoplasm. Plasma cell neoplasms can vary widely in histologic appearance from epithelioid to plasmacytoid to sarcomatoid; however, CD138 will stain all of these histologic appearances. Metastatic PEComa and melanoma can have prominent nucleoli but neither these nor the other answer choices would be CD138 positive.

13. **(a) Chondroblastoma**

The clinical history is consistent with chondroblastoma: a young patient with a long bone epiphyseal lesion that has a sclerotic rim. Histologically, the presence of mononuclear cells admixed with giant cells (blue arrow) and regions of light pink hyalinized matrix (black arrow), so-called fibrochondroid matrix, are diagnostic of chondroblastoma. Nonossifying fibroma is centered in the metaphysis and does not contain a hyalinized matrix. Giant cell tumor of bone is an epiphyseal lesion but would not show fibrochondroid matrix. Aneurysmal bone cyst is a metaphyseal lesion and can show osteoid but not fibrochondroid matrix. Chondromyxoid fibroma is a metaphyseal lesion.

14. **(c) McCune-Albright syndrome**

This lesion is polyostotic fibrous dysplasia from the curvilinear trabeculae, the bland eosinophilic intervening spindled cells, and the lack of osteoblastic rimming (the bland spindled cells abutting the bone are not osteoblasts, blue arrow). Polyostotic fibrous dysplasia is seen in McCune-Albright syndrome, a syndrome characterized by endocrine abnormalities (consistent with precocious puberty), café au lait spots, and polyostotic fibrous dysplasia. The other answer choices are not associated with polyostotic fibrous dysplasia.

15. **(b) Translocation involving 17p13.2**

This is an aneurysmal bone cyst with the typical blood filled spaces (black arrow), bland fibroblasts without cytologic atypia, giant cells (blue arrow), and new bone deposition (red arrow). 66% of aneurysmal bone cysts are associated with translocations of chromosomal region 17p13.2. T(11;22) is associated with Ewing's sarcoma and desmoplastic small round blue cell tumor neither of which would feature giant cells and blood filled spaces. T(X;18) is associated with synovial sarcoma which would not show new bone deposition or giant cells. Complex cytogenetic changes can be seen in undifferentiated pleomorphic sarcoma which has far more atypia.

16. **(c) Synovial lipomatosis**

The image shows a proliferation of adipocytes (black arrow) next to a synovial lining (blue arrow). The adipocytes are expanding the synovial space, leading to the villous synovial projection seen here and in most cases of synovial lipomatosis also known as lipoma arborescens. Angiolipoma would have thrombi in the vessels. Spindle cell lipoma would feature a spindled population. Angiomyolipoma would feature a smooth muscle component. Hemangioma would not explain the proliferation of mature adipocytes in the sub-synovial space.

17. **(e) S-100**

This is a case of Langerhans cell histiocytosis. This 10-year-old patient is within the predicted age range of Langerhans cell histiocytosis (5-15 years old). The histology shows occasional multilobated or irregularly shaped nuclei (Langerhans cells, black arrow) as well as a prominent eosinophilic infiltrate (red arrow). These Langerhans cells often show a grooved chromatin pattern. Langerhans cell histiocytosis stains strongly for CD1a, S-100, and langerin. S-100 is the only one included in the answer choices. CD30 and CD15 would highlight a case of Hodgkin's lymphoma which is not likely as no true Reed Sternberg cells are seen and Hodgkin's would be rare in a patient this young.

18. **(c) Hemosiderotic synovitis**

The clinical history of a patient with hemophilia and the histologic findings of abundant hemosiderin (red arrow) and small arterioles (blue arrow) favor hemosiderotic synovitis. There are no giant cells present that would be seen with PVNS. Intrasynovial hemangioma could be associated with hemosiderin deposition but would show a proliferation of capillary or cavernous sized vessels. Loose body would show cartilage and bone. Malignant melanoma would show atypical tumor cells.

CHAPTER 8

Small Round Blue Cell Tumors

1. An 80-year-old man with a distant history of resected colon cancer has diffuse mediastinal adenopathy with liver metastases. A liver biopsy shows the findings to the right. Tumor cells are positive for synaptophysin and chromogranin. What is the correct diagnosis?
   - (a) Hepatoblastoma
   - (b) Neuroblastoma
   - (c) Small lymphocytic lymphoma
   - (d) Recurrent colon cancer
   - (e) Metastatic small cell carcinoma

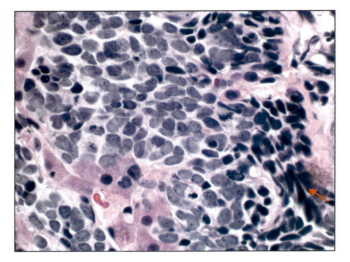

2. A 20-year-old man has a rapidly growing thigh mass with the histology shown. Which of the translocations is most likely present?
   - (a) PAX3-FKHR
   - (b) EWS-FlI1
   - (c) TFE3-ASPL
   - (d) EWS-WT1
   - (e) PDGFB-COL1A1

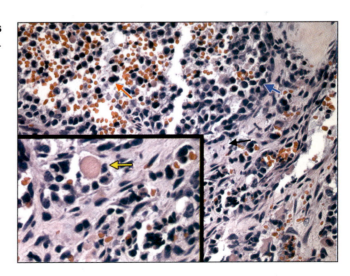

3. **A 6-month-old girl has leukocoria and the lesion depicted to the right. What is the correct diagnosis?**
   (a) Ewing's sarcoma
   (b) Neuroblastoma
   (c) Retinoblastoma
   (d) Small lymphocytic lymphoma
   (e) Melanoma

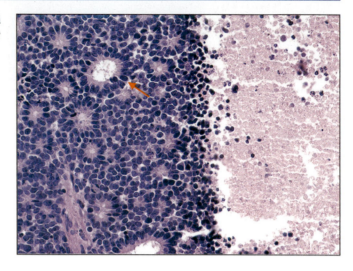

4. **A 14-year-old female has back pain and a 5.1 cm left mediastinal mass extending from the left hilar region through the aorticopulmonary window and more superiorly into the apex of the left lung, abutting the left pulmonary artery. Tumor cells stain positively for AE1/AE3, WT1, and exhibit perinuclear dot-like staining for desmin. A t(11;22) translocation is present. What is the correct diagnosis?**
   (a) Alveolar rhabdomyosarcoma
   (b) Metastatic Wilm's tumor, blastemal predominant
   (c) Desmoplastic small round blue cell tumor
   (d) Ewing's sarcoma
   (e) Metastatic carcinoma

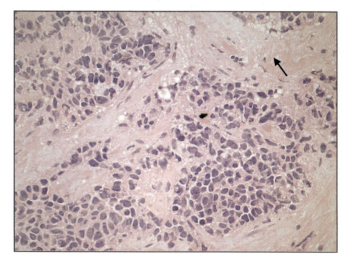

5. **A 71-year-old man has a 2 cm left forearm skin lesion and no additional lesions on a whole body scan. What stain most likely highlights these cells?**
   (a) CD99
   (b) Fli-1
   (c) CK20
   (d) CD45
   (e) TTF1-1

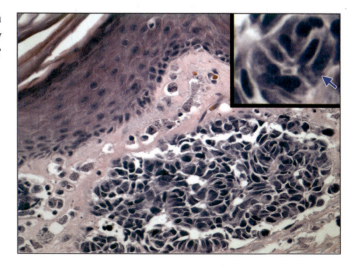

6. **A 22-month-old girl has an 8 cm partially calcified pelvic mass attached to the right ovary. Histology from the mass is shown to the right. What is the correct diagnosis?**
   (a) Neuroblastoma
   (b) Ganglioneuroma
   (c) Ganglioneuroblastoma
   (d) Pheochromocytoma
   (e) Wilm's tumor

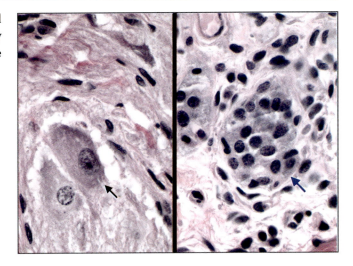

7. **A 2.5-month-old boy has a 3.4 cm heterogeneous enhancing mass in the right maxillary alveolar ridge extending into the right maxillary sinus and the right nasal cavity. It encases several teeth and abuts the right infraorbital foramen. What is the correct diagnosis?**
   (a) Metastatic neuroblastoma
   (b) Desmoplastic small round blue cell tumor
   (c) Melanotic neuroectodermal tumor of infancy
   (d) Malignant melanoma
   (e) Alveolar rhabdomyosarcoma

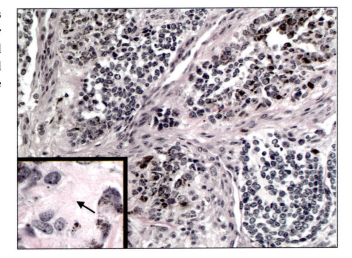

8. **A 19-year-old female has a lytic right tibial diaphyseal lesion with an onion skin appearance radiologically. Stains for CD99 and Fli-1 are positive while a tdt stain is negative. Myogenin and MyoD1 are negative. What is the correct diagnosis?**
   (a) Ewing's sarcoma
   (b) Acute lymphoblastic leukemia
   (c) Neuroblastoma
   (d) Desmoplastic small round blue cell tumor
   (e) Osteosarcoma, small cell variant

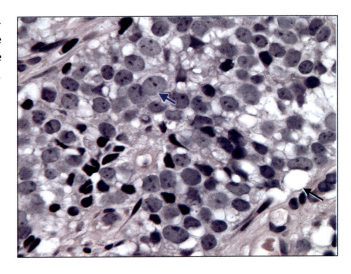

9. A 6-year-old has multiple bone metastases and cauda equina metastatic involvement by a primary tumor depicted to the right. Imaging shows a posterior fossa mass. Tumor cells stain for NSE and synaptophysin. CD99 and desmin are negative. What is the most likely primary tumor?
   (a) Ewing's sarcoma
   (b) Desmoplastic small round blue cell tumor
   (c) Neuroblastoma
   (d) Merkel cell carcinoma
   (e) Medulloblastoma

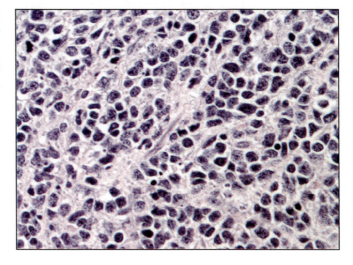

10. A 4-year-old boy presented with multiple petechiae and a bone marrow biopsy was diagnostic of metastatic disease. On closer examination the patient is found to have a 1.5 cm mobile mass in the deep left calf depicted here. What is the correct diagnosis?
    (a) Alveolar rhabdomyosarcoma
    (b) Acute myeloid leukemia
    (c) Burkitt's lymphoma
    (d) Neuroblastoma
    (e) Embryonal rhabdomyosarcoma

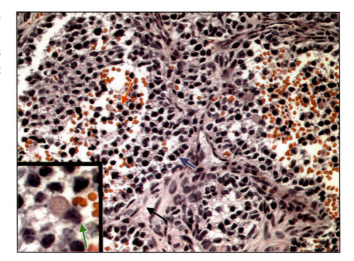

11. A 2-month-old child has a 4 cm heterogeneously enhancing lesion of the kidney right upper pole and adrenal, diffusely infiltrating the liver. Tumor cells stain positively for chromogranin and synaptophysin. Serum AFP is not elevated. What is the correct diagnosis?
    (a) Hepatoblastoma, anaplastic variant
    (b) Neuroblastoma
    (c) Desmoplastic small round blue cell tumor
    (d) Alveolar rhabdomyosarcoma
    (e) Metastatic small cell carcinoma

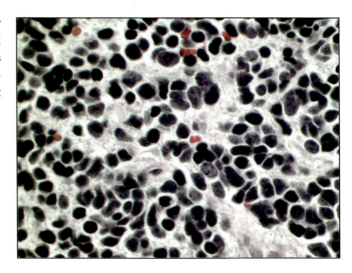

12. **An 18-year-old male has a right buttock 8 cm soft tissue mass shown to the right that stains positively for CD99 and Fli-1. Myogenin and myoD1 are negative. What translocation is most likely present?**
    (a) T(11;22)
    (b) T(2;13)
    (c) T(9;22)
    (d) T(x;18)
    (e) T(12;22)

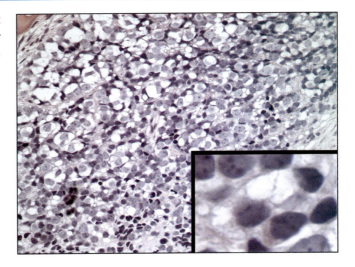

13. **A 6-month-old boy has a mass at the roof of his mouth that is depicted to the right. What stain highlights the pigmented cells?**
    (a) Cytokeratin
    (b) Chromogranin
    (c) CEA
    (d) Desmin
    (e) S-100

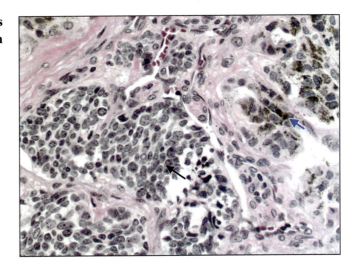

14. **A 4-year-old female has a 3.5 cm heterogeneously enhancing mass in her right temporal bone extending into the external auditory canal. What is the correct diagnosis?**
    (a) Merkel cell carcinoma
    (b) Mycosis fungoides
    (c) Embryonal rhabdomyosarcoma
    (d) Myxoid liposarcoma
    (e) Mesenchymal chondrosarcoma

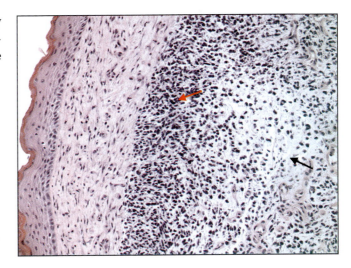

15. **An 11-month-old male infant has a solid heterogeneous 7 cm right renal mass by ultrasound with the histology shown to the right that stains for WT-1. What is the correct diagnosis?**
    - (a) Desmoplastic small round blue cell tumor
    - (b) Wilm's tumor, blastemal predominant
    - (c) Ewing's sarcoma
    - (d) Alveolar rhabdomyosarcoma, solid variant
    - (e) Neuroblastoma

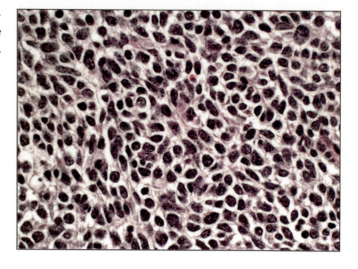

16. **A 70-year-old man has a WBC of 190,000 and a bone marrow biopsy shows the findings to the right. What stain will most likely highlight these cells?**
    - (a) WT-1
    - (b) CD99
    - (c) Fli-1
    - (d) CD23
    - (e) CD138

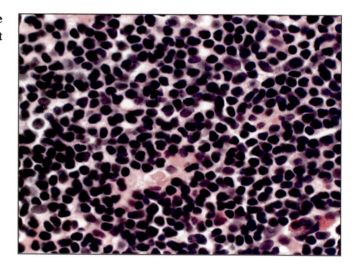

17. **An 8-year-old female has a deep left lower leg rapidly growing mass. Tumor cells display nuclear positivity for myoD1. What is the correct diagnosis?**
    - (a) Small lymphocytic lymphoma
    - (b) Alveolar rhabdomyosarcoma
    - (c) Ewing's sarcoma
    - (d) Desmoplastic small round blue cell tumor
    - (e) Merkel cell carcinoma

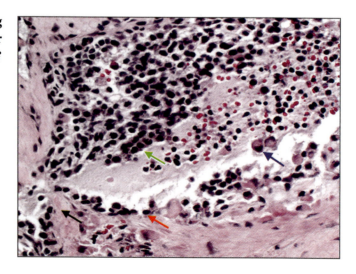

18. A 24-year-old female has pain and a circumscribed, calcified soft tissue mass in her left leg by radiology. The cellular areas (blue arrow) stain positively for CD99 while the less cellular areas (red arrow) are highlighted by S-100. What is the correct diagnosis?

   (a) Ewing's sarcoma
   (b) Neuroblastoma
   (c) Alveolar rhabdomyosarcoma
   (d) Desmoplastic small round blue cell tumor
   (e) Mesenchymal chondrosarcoma

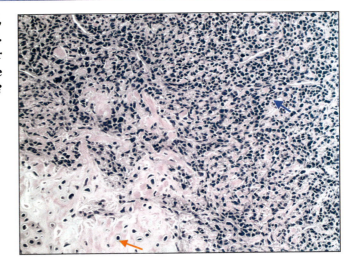

ANSWERS

1. **(e) Metastatic small cell carcinoma**

   The tumor shows sheets of small round blue cells some of which display nuclear moulding to such a degree that nuclear smudging is seen (red arrow). Nuclear moulding and smudging are highly suspicious for metastatic small cell carcinoma. The clinical history of mediastinal adenopathy also points towards small cell carcinoma. This patient is outside of the age range of hepatoblastoma and neuroblastoma which occur before the age of 5 and 1, respectively. Small lymphocytic lymphoma would not show nuclear smudging. Recurrent colon cancer would likely show glandular architecture.

2. **(a) PAX3-FKHR**

   PAX3-FKHR is associated with alveolar rhabdomyosarcoma. This tumor often presents as a rapidly growing mass in the extremities of a young person. Thick fibrous septae (black arrow) are seen separating pseudo-alveolar spaces containing discohesive small round blue tumor cells (red arrow) and small round blue tumor cells hugging the fibrous lining (blue arrow). Occasional rhabdomyoblasts with eccentric nuclei and abundant eosinophilic cytoplasm can be seen (yellow arrow). EWS-FLI1 is associated with Ewing's sarcoma and EWS-WT1 is associated with desmoplastic small round blue cell tumor, both small round blue cell tumors without pseudo-alveolar histology. TFE3-ASPL is associated with alveolar soft part sarcoma which would have cells with abundant eosinophilic cytoplasm, not small round blue cells. PDGFB-COL1A1 is associated with dermatofibrosarcoma protuberans which would show storiform not alveolar architecture.

3. **(c) Retinoblastoma**

   The histology depicts a sheet of small round blue cells with occasional tubule formation displaying peripheral palisading (Flexner-Wintersteiner rosettes, red arrow) and necrosis. These findings are typical for retinoblastoma and leukocoria is a main clinical finding in many cases. Ewing's sarcoma would not feature Flexner-Wintersteiner rosettes or Homer-Wright rosettes. Neuroblastoma could show Homer Wright rosettes but not Flexner-Wintersteiner rosettes. Homer Wright rosettes feature palisaded cells around a neuropil core without a central clear lumen. Small lymphocytic lymphoma and melanoma would not show rosettes.

4. **(c) Desmoplastic small round blue cell tumor**

   Desmoplastic small round blue cell tumor (DSRBCT) shows the histologic findings of groups of small angulated blue cells with minimal cytoplasm separated by thick fibrous bands (black arrow) shown in the image. A mediastinal location is atypical for this most commonly abdominal or pelvic tumor. Nevertheless, WT1 staining, desmin perinuclear dot-like staining, and the presence of the t(11;22) translocation narrow the differential diagnosis to desmoplastic small round blue cell tumor. T(11;22) can also be seen in Ewing's sarcoma but Ewing's sarcoma would stain negatively for WT1. Metastatic Wilm's tumor, alveolar rhabdomyosarcoma, and metastatic carcinoma would not show this characteristic translocation.

5. **(c) CK20**

   This is a Merkel cell carcinoma. Diagnostically contributory features include the age of the patient (adult), the dermal location of the lesion, the presence of small round blue cells, and the prominent nuclear moulding (blue arrow). CK20 highlights Merkel cell carcinoma in a perinuclear dot-like fashion. CD99 and Fli-1 would highlight Ewing's sarcoma/PNET; however Ewing's sarcoma occurs between the ages of 5–40 years and the dermis would be an atypical site for Ewing's sarcoma. CD45 would highlight a lymphoma but nuclear moulding to this degree would not be seen in lymphoma. TTF-1 would be positive in metastatic small cell carcinoma which can also show nuclear moulding; however, in the absence of any additional lesions on whole body imaging, Merkel cell carcinoma is the most likely diagnosis.

6. **(c) Ganglioneuroblastoma**

   Ganglioneuroblastoma is a subtype of neuroblastoma in which mature ganglion cells with abundant cytoplasm, eccentric nuclei, and prominent nucleoli (black arrow) are seen in some parts of the tumor and other parts of the tumor show nests of immature "small round blue" cells (blue arrow). Ganglioneuroblastoma is more differentiated and generally has a better prognosis than neuroblastoma. Ganglioneuroma would have ganglion cells and Schwann cells, without the primitive cell population seen here. Neuroblastoma would not feature ganglion cells. Pheochromocytoma and Wilm's tumor would not show ganglion cells.

7. **(c) Melanotic neuroectodermal tumor of infancy**

Melanotic neuroectodermal tumor of infancy most often occurs in the maxilla of infants. Histologically, nests of small round blue cells can be seen with occasional neurofibrillary material (black arrow). The nests are lined by or associated with large pigmented epithelioid cells. Metastatic neuroblastoma, desmoplastic small round blue cell tumor, and alveolar rhabdomyosarcoma are all small round blue cell tumors that can affect children and young adults but none would have large pigmented epithelioid cells. Malignant melanoma would not show neurofibrillary material and would have atypical large cells, not an intermixed small round blue cell population.

8. **(a) Ewing's sarcoma**

Radiologically, this tumor shows a lytic long bone diaphyseal lesion with onion skinning, all features consistent with Ewing's sarcoma. The patient's age of 19 is in the Ewing's afflicted age range of 5–20 years of age. Histologically, the image shows findings consistent with Ewing's sarcoma: sheets of small round blue cells some of which display cytoplasmic clearing (black arrow) and dispersed chromatin with small nucleoli (blue arrow). Acute lymphoblastic leukemia also shows sheets of small round cells with dispersed chromatin and many stain positively for CD99 and Fli-1. Some cases of acute lymphoblastic leukemia also stain negatively for CD45, increasing diagnostic confusion. Tdt negativity and the radiologic onion skin appearance rule against acute lymphoblastic leukemia. This patient is too old for neuroblastoma which typically occurs in patients younger than one year old. Desmopastic small round blue cell tumor often presents as a peritoneal tumor and a bone lesion presentation would be atypical. Osteosarcoma, small cell variant would feature osteoid production.

9. **(e) Medulloblastoma**

This is a medulloblastoma showing groups of small round blue cells. CD99 and desmin negativity rule out Ewing's sarcoma and desmoplastic small round blue cell tumor, respectively. Given the presence of a posterior fossa mass, the most likely site of medulloblastoma, the metastases are likely due to it.

10. **(a) Alveolar rhabdomyosarcoma**

As depicted in the image, alveolar rhabdomyosarcoma features fibrous septae (black arrow) surrounding quasi-alveolar spaces which contain dyscohesive nests of cells (red arrow). The alveolar spaces are lined by tumor cells (blue arrow). Scattered rhabdomyoblasts with abundant eosinophilic cytoplasm and eccentric nuclei can be seen (green arrow). Alveolar rhabdomyosarcoma is a small round blue cell tumor and the tumor cells have high N:C ratios with round nuclei. The other answer choices lack the quasi-alveolar growth pattern seen here.

11. **(b) Neuroblastoma**

This tumor shows small round blue cells almost devoid of cytoplasm with high N/C ratios, consistent with neuroblastoma. This tumor occurs predominantly in patients younger than 1 year old and often appears associated with the adrenal gland, as in this case. Synaptophysin and chromogranin are positive in neuroblastoma. Hepatoblastoma occurs in patients younger than 5 years of age and can have a small round blue cell appearance but would feature an elevated AFP. Desmoplastic small round blue cell tumor also causes an abdominal mass but occurs most often in patients between the ages of 15–35 years and would be negative for chromogranin and synaptophysin. The patient is too young to have metastatic small cell carcinoma. Chromogranin and synaptophysin will be negative in alveolar rhabdomyosarcoma.

12. **(a) T(11;22)**

Sheets of small round blue cells are seen, some of which have clear cytoplasm. Some of the cells display dispersed chromatin and some show small nucleoli. These histologic findings are consistent with Ewing's sarcoma. Additionally, the patient's age of 18 (between 5 and 20 years old) and tumor immunoprofile showing CD99 and Fli-1 positivity also support Ewing's sarcoma. Ewing's sarcoma has been linked to the EWS-Fli1 translocation, t(11;22), which can be seen in the vast majority of cases. T(2;13) is seen in alveolar rhabdomyosarcoma which is ruled out by a lack of myogenin and myoD1 stianing. Myxoid chondrosarcoma shows a t(9;22) translocation but this case shows no fibrous septae or myxoid background. T(x;18) is found in synovial sarcoma which would typically have a more spindled appearance, less dispersed chromatin, and stain negatively for Fli-1. T(12;22) is seen in clear cell sarcoma which is typically CD99 negative.

13. **(a) Cytokeratin**

This is a melanotic neuroectodermal tumor of infancy, characterized by a small round blue cell population (black arrow) and a larger pigmented epithelioid population (blue arrow). The small round blue cell component is often nested as in this image. The large pigmented cells in this lesion are always positive for cytokeratin. These cells are negative for the remaining markers.

14. **(c) Embryonal rhabdomyosarcoma**

This is an embryonal rhabdomyosarcoma with a dermal proliferation of immature "small round blue cells" displaying alternating hypercellular (red arrow) and hypocellular, myxoid (black arrow) regions. Some embryonal rhabdomyosarcoma cases can show rhabdomyoblastic differentiation; however, this case is entirely immature with no rhabdomyoblasts. Merkel cell carcinoma and mycosis fungoides do not feature alternating hypercellular and hypocellular areas. Myxoid liposarcoma could show more hypercellular regions if there were a round cell component but for that diagnosis we would need more prominent delicate vasculature. Mesenchymal chondrosarcoma would show some cartilaginous differentiation intermixed with small round blue cells.

15. **(b) Wilm's tumor, blastemal predominant**

Wilm's tumor shows immature blastemal cells occasionally with an epithelial component or an anaplastic component. This tumor is blastemal predominant, composed solely of immature small cells with high N:C rations. The renal location and age of the patient make Wilm's tumor and neuroblastoma (adrenal, usually) higher on the differential diagnosis. Neuroblastoma rarely stains for WT-1. Desmoplastic small round blue cell tumor would stain for WT1 but the age of the patient, 11 months, is too young for desmoplastic small round blue cell tumor that typically occurs in patients between 15 and 35 years of age. Additionally, desmoplastic small round blue cell tumor would show fibrous septae. Ewing's sarcoma would be negative for WT-1. A renal primary focus would be an unusual presentation for alveolar rhabdomyosarcoma which often occurs in the deep soft tissues of the extremities and shows fibrous septae dividing discohesive small round blue cells.

16. **(d) CD23**

This is small lymphocytic lymphoma/chronic lymphocytic leukemia (SLL/CLL). The clinical history of a markedly elevated white blood count in an elderly patient suggests the diagnosis. Histologically, discohesive monotonous small round blue cells are seen as is shown in the image. In most cases CD23 is positive and CD138 is negative. WT-1 would be positive in blastemal predominant Wilm's tumor or desmoplastic small round blue cell tumor; the patient is out of the correct age range for both these tumors. CD99 and Fli-1 would be positive in Ewing's sarcoma which would occur in children or young adults; it would not feature leukocytosis.

17. **(b) Alveolar rhabdomyosarcoma**

Alveolar rhabdomyosarcoma, a sarcoma with a preference for the extremity soft tissue of children near the ages of 7–9, exhibits discohesive small round blue cells (green arrow) separated by fibrovascular septae (black arrow). The cells line the septae (red arrow) and occasional dyscohesive rhabdomyoblasts with abundant eosinophilic cytoplasm and eccentric nuclei can be seen (blue arrow). Myogenin and myoD1 nuclear positivity is present in most cases. Ewing's sarcoma and desmoplastic small round blue cell tumor are negative for myoD1. Small lymphocytic lymphoma and merkel cell carcinoma would not have fibrovascular septae.

18. **(e) Mesenchymal chondrosarcoma**

This tumor is a mesenchymal chondrosarcoma because it displays cartilaginous foci (red arrow) immediately adjacent to a small round blue cell tumor (blue arrow). Mesenchymal chondrosarcoma is not uncommonly found as a soft tissue primary. The small round blue cells stain positively for CD99 while the cartilaginous region stains for S-100. Ewing's sarcoma would show CD99 positivity but cartilage is not a feature of it. Neuroblastoma, alveolar rhabdomyosarcoma, and desmoplastic small round blue cell tumor should not show cartilaginous differentiation.

CHAPTER 9

Joint and Bone Lesions with Giant Cells

1. **A 31-year-old female has a slow growing left knee mass. Radiology shows a well-circumscribed soft tissue mass. What is the correct diagnosis?**
   (a) Benign giant cell tumor of tendon sheath
   (b) Nonossifying fibroma
   (c) Giant cell reparative granuloma
   (d) Malignant giant cell tumor of tendon sheath
   (e) Pseudogout

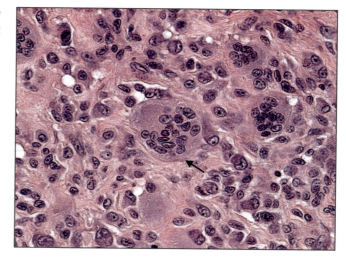

2. **A 65-year-old female has an anterior right knee mass. Imaging shows a 3.8 cm enhancing well-circumscribed mass in the vastus medialis muscle with no intra-articular or intraosseous extension. What is the correct diagnosis?**
   (a) Fibroma of tendon sheath
   (b) Malignant tenosynovial giant cell tumor
   (c) Synovial sarcoma
   (d) Benign tenosynovial giant cell tumor
   (e) Soft tissue giant cell tumor of low malignant potential

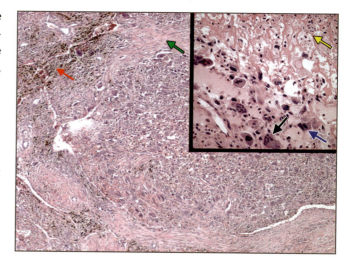

3. **A well-circumscribed distal femoral lesion is found incidentally in a 16-year-old boy. The lesion has a sclerotic rim and is metaphyseal. Histology from the lesion is shown to the right. The patient has also been having elbow pain recently and has multiple coffee-colored lesions diffusely involving his skin. What syndrome does he most likely suffer from?**
   (a) Neurofibromatosis 1
   (b) Neurofibromatosis 2
   (c) Tuberous sclerosis
   (d) Jaffe-Campanacci syndrome
   (e) Sturge-Weber syndrome

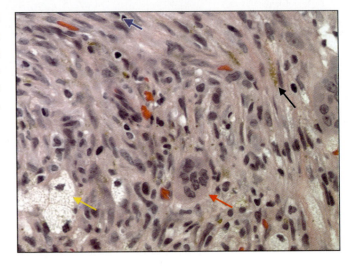

4. **A 22-year-old female has a 3 cm proximal tibial lucent lesion involving the epiphysis. Histology of the lesion is shown to the right. Based on the well-established prognosis of these tumors, what will be the most likely treatment approach?**
   (a) Chemotherapy alone
   (b) Radiation alone
   (c) Surgery, chemotherapy, and radiation
   (d) Surgery alone
   (e) Chemotherapy and radiation

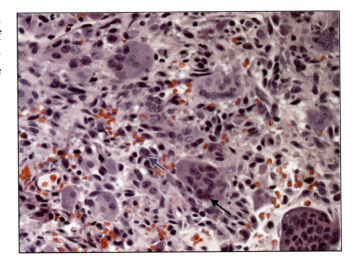

5. **A 52-year-old man has a knee MRI showing synovial based masses and magnetic susceptibility artifacts on a gradient echo sequence. Histology from one of the masses is shown to the right. What is the correct diagnosis?**
   (a) PVNS
   (b) Melanotic schwannoma
   (c) Synovial hemangioma
   (d) Tenosynovial giant cell tumor, localized type
   (e) Metastatic melanoma

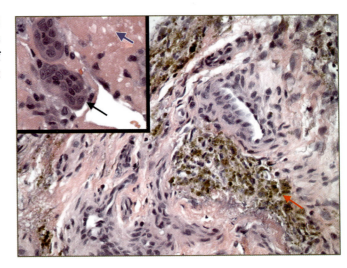

6. A 37-year-old man has had knee pain for several years and imaging shows a circumscribed nodule measuring 4 cm in the left knee joint posterior to the posterior cruciate ligament. What is the correct diagnosis?

(a) PVNS
(b) Tenosynovial giant cell tumor, localized form
(c) Tenosynovial giant cell tumor, diffuse form
(d) Nonossifying fibroma
(e) Pleomorphic undifferentiated sarcoma

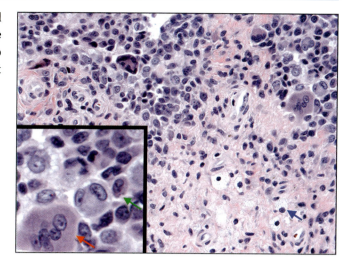

7. A 48-year-old male has had several years of worsening left hip pain and imaging shows a left femoral head epiphyseal lytic lesion. Histology from the lesion is shown to the right. What is the correct diagnosis?

(a) Hibernoma
(b) Metastatic chromophobe renal cell carcinoma
(c) Clear cell chondrosarcoma
(d) Chondroblastic osteosarcoma
(e) PEComa

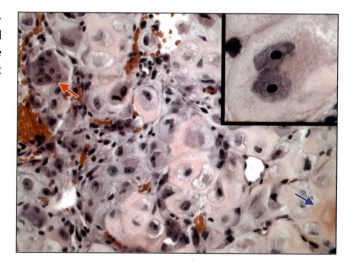

8. A 16-year-old boy has a 2 cm right femoral epiphysis lesion with a sclerotic rim. Histology from the lesion is depicted to the right. What histologic finding, found in approximately one third of cases but not in this case, is the most specific for this lesion?

(a) Giant cells mixed with mononuclear cells
(b) Intravascular calcifications
(c) Giant cell calcifications
(d) Pericellular chicken-wire calcifications
(e) Psammoma bodies

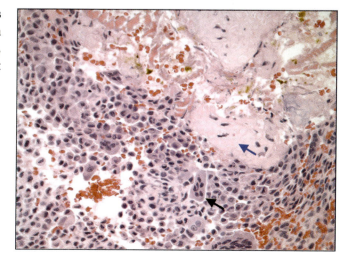

9. **A 24-year-old female has a partially cystic, partially solid left lateral femur epiphyseal lesion. What is the correct diagnosis?**
   (a) Aneurysmal bone cyst
   (b) Unicameral bone cyst
   (c) Giant cell tumor of bone
   (d) Chondroblastoma
   (e) Undifferentiated pleomorphic sarcoma, giant-cell variant

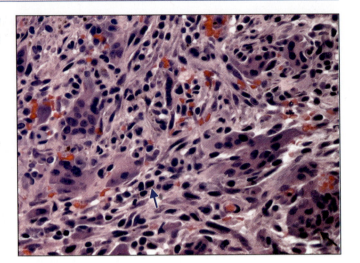

1. **(a) Benign giant cell tumor of tendon sheath**

   The radiologic appearance of a knee-region well-circumscribed soft tissue mass and the histologic features of numerous giant cells (black arrow) and cytologically similar mononuclear cells with no cytologic atypia are consistent with benign giant cell tumor of tendon sheath. Nonossifying fibroma and giant cell reparative granuloma would be in bone, not soft tissue. Malignant giant cell tumor of tendon sheath would show cytologic atypia, mitotic activity, or necrosis. Pseudogout can show giant cells but would also show rhomboid crystals.

2. **(b) Malignant tenosynovial giant cell tumor**

   This is a tenosynovial giant cell tumor because of its juxtaarticular location, its nodular architecture created by thick fibrous strands (green arrow), its hemosiderin deposition (red arrow), and the abundance of multinucleated giant cells (inset, black arrow). Cytologic features of malignancy include markedly atypical cells (blue arrow) and tumor-type necrosis (yellow arrow). Malignant tenosynovial giant cell tumor is a very rare disease but it best fits these clinical and histologic findings. The other answer choices would not have the malignant features seen here.

3. **(d) Jaffe-Campanacci syndrome**

   The clinical description of a teenage boy with a metaphyseal well-circumscribed lesion with a sclerotic rim is suggestive of nonossifying fibroma. The histologic image supports the diagnosis with several hallmarks of nonossifying fibroma displayed: hemosiderin laden macrophages (black arrow); monotonous spindled cells in fascicles (blue arrow); giant cells (red arrow); and foam cells (yellow arrow). The presence of the café au lait skin spots along with a nonossifying fibroma is most consistent with Jaffe-Campanacci syndrome. This syndrome is rare and can also feature mental retardation. The other answer choices are syndromes with characteristic skin lesions; however, none but Jaffe-Campanacci syndrome is associated with nonossifying fibromas.

4. **(d) Surgery alone**

   This is a giant cell tumor of bone displaying the classic demographic (young female), a classic site (proximal tibia, epiphyseal), and the well-established histologic features of the lesion, abundant multinucleated cells (black arrow) and uninucleated cells (blue arrow) which share an identical cytologic appearance. These tumors are considered locally aggressive with minimal metastatic potential. Rare pulmonary metastatic cases have been reported; however, even in these cases, the metastases have been self-limiting or have a very indolent clinical course. For this reason, the primary tumor and recurrences are treated surgically with no role for chemotherapy. Radiation therapy can be used for lesions that are not surgically accessible but it is not the first approach.

5. **(a) PVNS**

   PVNS displays the classic radiologic findings of synovial based masses and magnetic susceptibility artifacts on a gradient echo sequence. Epidemiologically, the knee is the most commonly affected joint. Histologically, it shows numerous giant cells (black arrow), occasional infarct type necrosis (blue arrow), and abundant hemosiderotic mononuclear cells (red arrow). The infarct type necrosis is a benign finding in this lesion and does not signify malignant change. Melanotic schwannoma and synovial hemangioma would not feature giant cells. Metastatic melanoma would show more nuclear pleomorphism and would not show those characteristic radiologic findings. Tenosynovial giant cell tumor, localized type, would be more nodular and circumscribed.

6. **(b) Tenosynovial giant cell tumor, localized form**

   This tenosynovial giant cell tumor has a characteristic history of pain for several years. Epidemiologically, the finger is the most common site for this lesion but other joints can be affected. Histologically, numerous giant cells are seen (red arrow) surrounded by cytologically similar mononuclear cells (green arrow) in a nodular, circumscribed arrangement. Scattered foam cells (blue arrow) can be seen associated with localized giant cell tumor. PVNS, also known as tenosynovial giant cell tumor diffuse form, would show villous protrusions. The nodularity of the cell groups seen here is most consistent with the localized form of tenosynovial giant cell tumor. Nonossifying fibroma is a medullary, not articular, lesion. Undifferentiated pleomorphic sarcoma would show more atypia.

7. **(c) Clear cell chondrosarcoma**

Clear cell chondrosarcoma, which favors the epiphysis of long bones, displays chondrocytes with abundant clear to eosinophilic cytoplasm, at least focal osteoid formation (blue arrow), large nucleoli, and scattered multi-nucleated giant cells (red arrow), as seen in the image. Hibernoma would not have clear cytoplasm; the cytoplasm of hibernoma is either homogenously eosinophilic or multivacuolated. Metastatic chromophobe renal cell carcinoma could have an eosinophilic hue to the cytoplasm but osteoid and giant cells are not a feature of renal cell carcinoma. Osteosarcoma typically involves the metaphysis of long bones, not the epiphysis. PEComa can have cells with clear to eosinophilic cytoplasm, prominent nucleoli, and scattered giant cells. An initial presentation for PEComa in the bone would be rare; favored sites include the uterus and abdominal-peritoneal locations. Additionally, osteoid should not be seen in PEComa.

8. **(d) Pericellular chicken-wire calcifications**

Pericellular chicken-wire calcifications, not seen in this image, are seen in approximately one third of chondroblastoma cases. Though not sensitive, they are a specific finding for chondroblastoma. The age of the patient (teenage), the size of the lesion (less than 5 cm), the site (long bone epiphysis), and the radiologic presence of a sclerotic rim all support the diagnosis of chondroblastoma. Diagnostic histologic findings include the presence of giant cells (black arrow) and mononuclear cells adjoining a light pink fibrochondroid matrix (blue arrow). Giant cells mixed with mononuclear cells is not specific for chondroblastoma. The other answer choices are not associated with chondroblastoma.

9. **(c) Giant cell tumor of bone**

This is a giant cell tumor of bone. Diagnostic features include the presence of numerous multinucleated giant cells (black arrow) and mononucleated cells (blue arrow). Characteristic of this lesion, the nuclei in the giant cells have a very similar histologic appearance to those in the mono-nucleated cells. As in the question stem, this lesion favors the long bone epiphyses of young women. Aneurysmal bone cyst histologically would show cystic spaces filled with blood and would more typically present in a metaphyseal location. Unicameral bone cyst would feature a cyst lining. Chondroblastoma would show a fibrochondroid matrix or chicken wire calcifications which are not seen here. Undifferentiated pleomorphic sarcoma, giant-cell variant would show bizarre nuclei with marked cytologic atypia.

CHAPTER 10

Lesions Forming Bone and Cartilage

1. **A 21-year-old man fell while mowing his lawn and developed painful right knee swelling. An X-ray showed a metaphyseal fracture of the distal femur associated with a lytic metaphyseal lesion. What is the correct diagnosis?**
   (a) Conventional intramedullary osteosarcoma
   (b) Fibrous dysplasia
   (c) Osteoid osteoma
   (d) Parosteal osteosarcoma
   (e) Aneurysmal bone cyst

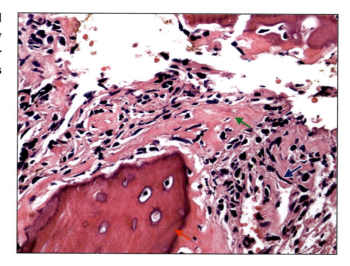

2. **A 10-year-old girl has a 10 cm left femoral lesion arising in the cortical portion of the proximal femoral diaphysis. The edge of the lesion shows a spiculated periosteal reaction with a Codman triangle. Representative histology is shown to the right. Not represented are regions of geographic necrosis seen elsewhere in the tumor. What is the correct diagnosis?**
   (a) Conventional osteosarcoma
   (b) High grade surface osteosarcoma
   (c) Parosteal osteosarcoma
   (d) Periosteal osteosarcoma
   (e) Desmoplastic fibroma

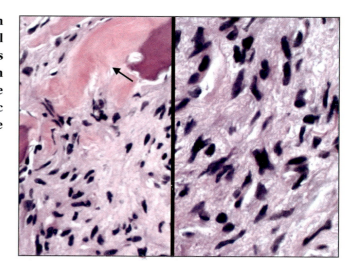

3. **An 18-year-old man has a 5 cm lesion involving the L3 vertebral body bone. Radiology shows a sclerotic bone rim surrounding the well-circumscribed lesion. His back pain is refractory to aspirin. The excisional specimen is shown to the right. What is the correct diagnosis?**
   (a) Osteoid osteoma
   (b) Osteosarcoma
   (c) Fibrous dysplasia
   (d) Osteofibrous dysplasia
   (e) Osteoblastoma

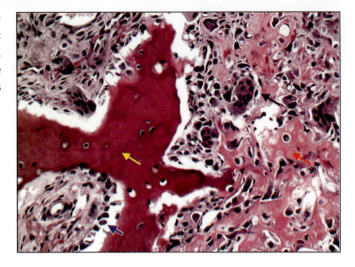

4. **A 67-year-old male has an enhancing mass measuring 7.8 cm in the right acetabulum with erosion of the right acetabulum and right superior pubic ramus. Radiology suggests central necrosis. An S-100 stain is seen on the right. An H&E stain of the region near the black arrow is expanded in the inset. What is the correct diagnosis?**
   (a) Conventional chondrosarcoma
   (b) High grade chondrosarcoma
   (c) Dedifferentiated chondrosarcoma
   (d) Undifferentiated sarcoma
   (e) Fibrosarcoma

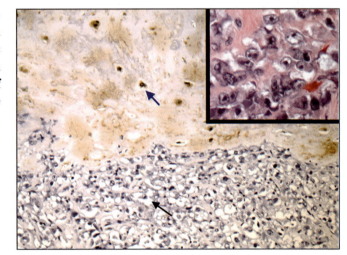

5. **A 55-year-old man has a lobular right proximal femur lesion with rim and septal enhancement. It is primarily intramedullary, measuring 13 cm craniocaudal. There is 8 cm of extraosseous extension with adjacent quadriceps edema. What is the correct diagnosis?**
   (a) Low grade intramedullary chondrosarcoma
   (b) High grade intramedullary chondrosarcoma
   (c) Enchondroma
   (d) Osteochondroma
   (e) Chondroblastic osteosarcoma

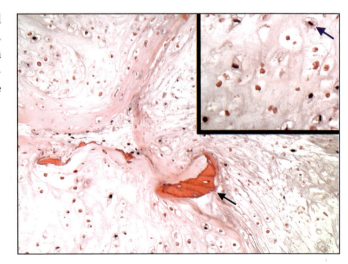

6. **A 35-year-old female has an ill-defined lucency with punctate calcifications in the left distal femur metaphysis. What is the correct diagnosis?**
   - (a) Enchondroma
   - (b) Osteochondroma
   - (c) Low grade chondrosarcoma
   - (d) High grade chondrosarcoma
   - (e) Periosteal osteosarcoma

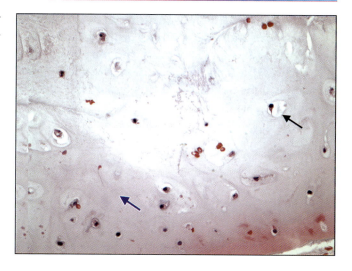

7. **A 17-year-old man with a history of left medial knee pain has a firm nodule over the left medial knee. Imaging shows a well-defined lesion in the medial proximal tibial metaphysis with no invasion into neighboring soft tissue. A biopsy of the lesion is shown to the right. What is the correct diagnosis?**
   - (a) Low grade chondrosarcoma
   - (b) Synovial chondromatosis
   - (c) Loose body
   - (d) Soft tissue chondroma
   - (e) Osteochondroma

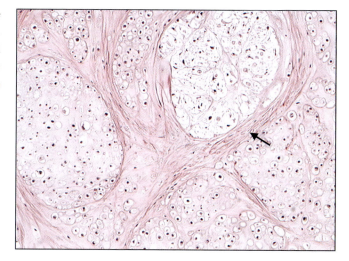

8. **An 80-year-old female has a right orbital 3.1 cm mass displacing the superior rectus muscle laterally and the globe anteriorly. Lesional tissue is depicted. What is the correct diagnosis?**
   - (a) Ossifying fibromyxoid tumor
   - (b) Chondroid syringoma
   - (c) Extraskeletal osteosarcoma
   - (d) Canalicular adenoma
   - (e) Retiform hemangioendothelioma

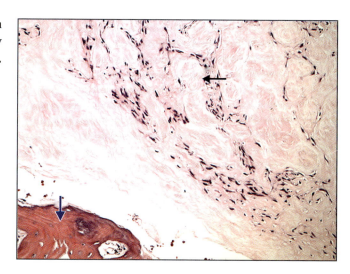

9. A 34-year-old female has a posterior distal femoral mass with the histology shown to the right. Imaging shows a 12 cm lobulated mass wrapping around the cortex of the femur. What is the approximate 5 year survival for patients with this tumor who receive optimal care?

(a) 100%
(b) 90%
(c) 60%
(d) 40%
(e) 20%

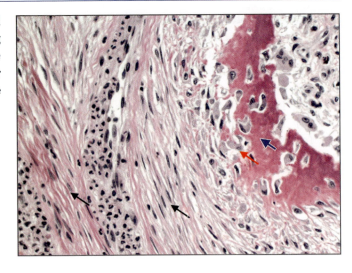

10. What is the most common site for the well-circumscribed 3 cm mass depicted to the right?

(a) Metaphysis of long bones
(b) Metaphysis of short bones
(c) Pelvis
(d) Epiphysis of long bones
(e) Diaphysis of long bones

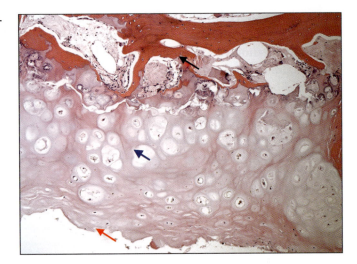

11. A healthy 30-year-old with no significant past medical history has a right proximal humerus medullary sclerotic mass that is incidentally found on routine imaging. The mass is excised and shown to the right. What is the correct diagnosis?

(a) Fracture callus
(b) Enostosis
(c) No diagnosis; benign bone
(d) Osteoradionecrosis
(e) Osteoblastoma

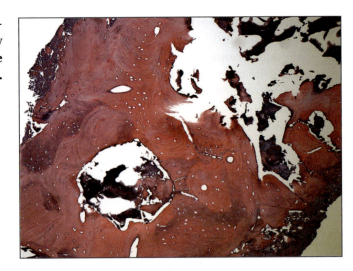

12. **A 12-year-old boy has a 1 cm right small finger mass that has been growing for the past few months. The histologic appearance of this mass is shown to the right. What is the correct diagnosis?**
    (a) Osteoblastoma
    (b) Osteoid osteoma
    (c) Fracture callus
    (d) Osteosarcoma
    (e) Aneurysmal bone cyst

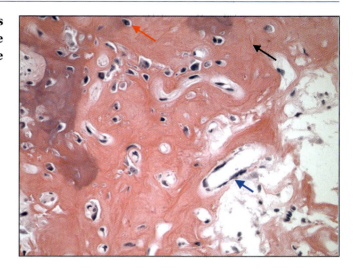

13. **A 33-year-old female has a 6 mm calcified cortical bony lesion near the right ethmoid bulla. Histology from the lesion is shown to the right. What is the correct diagnosis?**
    (a) Osteoid osteoma
    (b) Bone island
    (c) Osteoma
    (d) Benign bone
    (e) Osteoblastoma

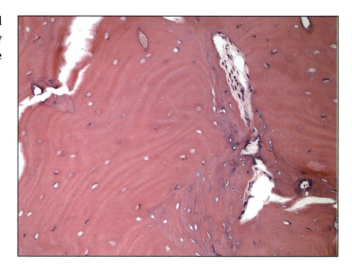

14. **Which of the following is not a subtype of the tumor shown to the right?**
    (a) Osteoblastic
    (b) Chondroblastic
    (c) Small cell
    (d) Large cell
    (e) Telangiectatic

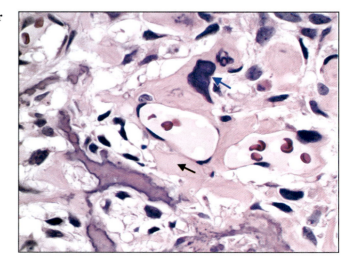

15. **A 7-year-old boy has bony growths in the left anterior 4ᵗʰ rib, the right scapula, the left proximal humerus, and the right clavicle. A right scapular biopsy is shown to the right. What syndrome does he most likely suffer from?**
    - (a) Gardner's syndrome
    - (b) Carney complex
    - (c) Multiple hereditary exostoses
    - (d) Maffucci syndrome
    - (e) Mazabraud's syndrome

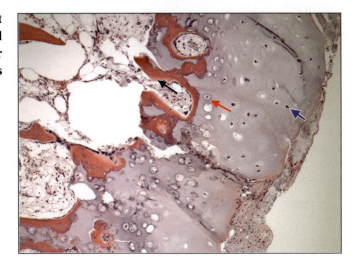

16. **A 23-year-old man has a lesion that shows heterogeneous uptake in the left distal femur. The lesion is depicted to the right. What is the correct diagnosis?**
    - (a) Angiosarcoma
    - (b) Undifferentiated pleomorphic sarcoma
    - (c) Telangiectatic osteosarcoma
    - (d) Osteosarcoma, small cell variant
    - (e) Aneurysmal bone cyst

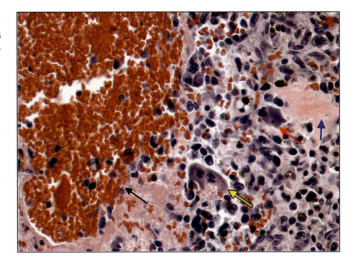

17. **An 8-year-old female has a 2.3 cm mass in the left jaw located in the mandibular ramus and invading into the mandible. What is the correct diagnosis?**
    - (a) Hemangiopericytoma
    - (b) Phosphaturic mesenchymal tumor
    - (c) Osteochondroma
    - (d) Myositis ossificans
    - (e) Chondroblastoma

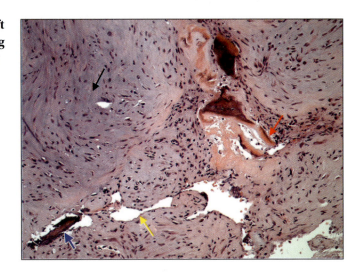

18. A 43-year-old woman has a recurrent 5 cm left buccal mass with a dumbbell shape displacing the buccinator muscle and impeding her ability to chew. The previous diagnosis was spindle cell lipoma. Lesional tissue is depicted. What is the correct diagnosis?

    (a) Well-differentiated liposarcoma
    (b) Spindle cell lipoma with osseous metaplasia and myxoid changes
    (c) Dedifferentiated liposarcoma
    (d) Well-differentiated osteosarcoma
    (e) Myxoid liposarcoma

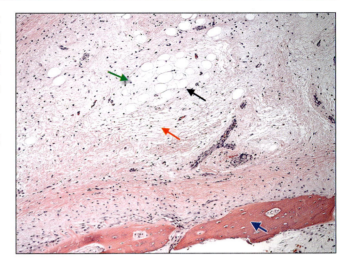

19. A 13-year-old girl has 4 weeks of pain in her left tibia. Imaging shows an intramedullary proximal left tibial lesion and 2 distal left tibia cortical lesions. Radiologically, none of the lesions shows aggressive characteristics. The histology to the right is representative of all lesions. What is the correct diagnosis?

    (a) Ollier's disease
    (b) Enchondroma
    (c) Chondroblastic osteosarcoma
    (d) Chondroblastoma
    (e) High grade chondrosarcoma

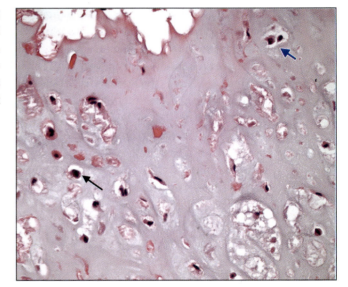

20. A 49-year-old man has a mass on his distal left index finger that has been present for several years. Radiology shows a 1 cm lesion superficially eroding cortical bone and overlying cortical sclerosis. No medullary involvement is seen. Microscopically, cartilaginous nodules are identified with the histologic appearance shown on the right. What is the correct diagnosis?

    (a) Periosteal chondrosarcoma
    (b) Enchondroma
    (c) Periosteal chondroma
    (d) Periosteal osteosarcoma
    (e) Synovial chondromatosis

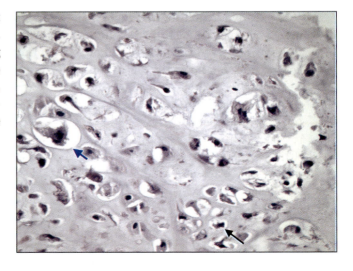

21. A 12-year-old girl has knee pain. Imaging shows a distal femoral meta-diaphyseal lesion with a permeative appearance. Periosteal reaction, sclerosis, cortical breakthrough, and ossification are seen. What is the correct diagnosis?
    (a) Chondroblastic osteosarcoma
    (b) Osteoblastic osteosarcoma
    (c) Small cell variant of osteosarcoma
    (d) Paget's disease
    (e) Intramedullary well-differentiated osteosarcoma

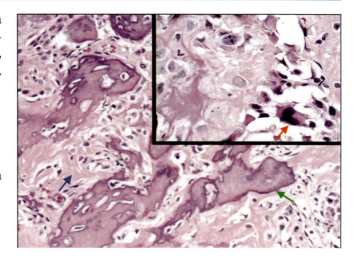

22. An 11-year-old girl has a 4.2 cm left iliac wing mass extending posteriorly into soft tissue to abut the gluteus maximus muscle. It displays a heterogeneous enhancement at the margin with no central enhancement. It invades the lateral part of sacrum as well. What is the correct diagnosis?
    (a) Chondrosarcoma
    (b) Chondroblastic osteosarcoma
    (c) Osteoblastic osteosarcoma
    (d) Oseoblastoma
    (e) Small cell osteosarcoma

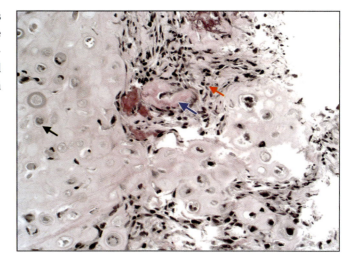

23. A 52-year-old female has a lobulated, heterogeneous 13 cm mass in the proximal tibial metaphysis. Imaging shows peripheral T2 enhancement and central nonenhancement, consistent with central necrosis. The lesion extends into the tibialis anterior muscle and into the popliteus muscle. What is the correct diagnosis?
    (a) Fibroblastic osteosarcoma
    (b) Chondroblastic osteosarcoma
    (c) Osteoid osteoma
    (d) Osteoblastoma
    (e) Fibrosarcoma

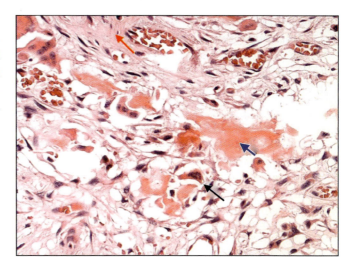

24. There is a well-circumscribed nodule near the left metatarsal head of a 68-year-old female. What is the correct diagnosis?

- (a) Osteoid osteoma
- (b) Chondroblastoma
- (c) Osteochondroma
- (d) Fibrous dysplasia
- (e) Reactive osteochondromatous proliferation

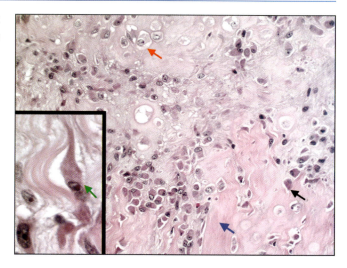

25. A 54-year-old female has throbbing pain localized to a right little finger swelling. MRI demonstrates a bone lesion involving up to 80% of the proximal phalanx. The differential diagnosis pre-excision includes enchondroma vs giant cell tumor of tendon sheath. What is the correct diagnosis?

- (a) Giant cell tumor of tendon sheath
- (b) Giant cell reparative granuloma
- (c) Fracture callus
- (d) Well-differentiated intramedullary osteosarcoma
- (e) Nonossifying fibroma

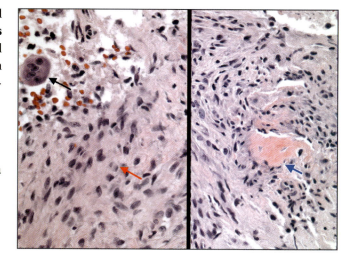

26. A large posterior tibial mass is found in a 38-year-old man with the histology shown to the right. The mass wraps around the tibia and the patient has noticed decreased knee mobility for the past year. What chromosomal change is most likely present?

- (a) Amplification of 12q13-15
- (b) Translocation involving 17p13
- (c) T(11;22)
- (d) T(12;15)
- (e) T(12;22)

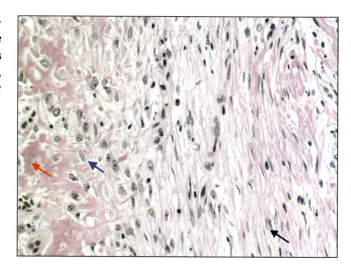

27. **A 50-year-old female has several months of lateral right right leg pain with proximal leg swelling after which a well-circumscribed mass was radiographically identified in the lateral calf. What is the correct diagnosis?**
    - (a) Myositis ossificans
    - (b) Extraskeletal osteosarcoma
    - (c) Chondrosarcoma
    - (d) Fibrosarcoma
    - (e) Nodular fasciitis

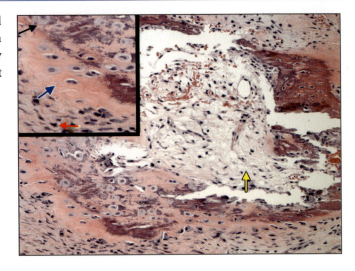

28. **A 47-year-old female has had a 4 cm right anterior knee mass for one year. What is the correct diagnosis?**
    - (a) Myxoid lipoma
    - (b) Fat necrosis
    - (c) Lipoma with osseous changes
    - (d) Chondroid lipoma
    - (e) Myxoid liposarcoma

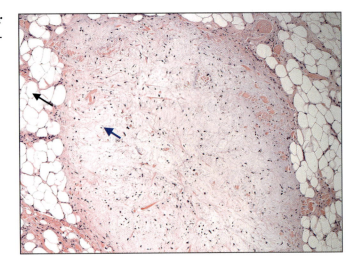

29. **A 19-year-old man has a lengthy history of limited left hip motion with associated pain. Imaging shows a pedunculated mass arising in the lesser trochanter measuring 4.4 cm There is mass effect on the obturator externus muscle. The underlying lesser trochanter is normal and there is no associated invasion of soft tissue. What is the correct diagnosis?**
    - (a) Chondrosarcoma
    - (b) Parosteal osteosarcoma
    - (c) Osteochondroma
    - (d) Osteoid osteoma
    - (e) Osteopetrosis

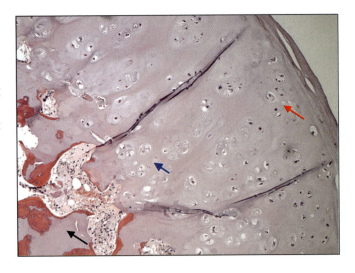

30. A 33-year-old woman has a distal left femur meta-physeal heterogeneous mass measuring 7.7 cm centered in the medulla but extending through the cortex. Extensive extraosseous edema and periosteal reaction is present. Histology from the resection is shown to the right. What is the correct diagnosis?

- (a) Low grade intramedullary osteosarcoma
- (b) Fibrous dysplasia
- (c) High grade surface osteosarcoma
- (d) Parosteal osteosarcoma
- (e) Periosteal osteosarcoma

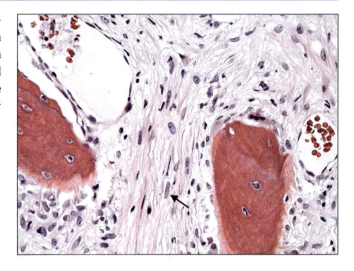

31. A 47-year-old female has multiple lytic painless medullary bone lesions. What is the correct diagnosis?

- (a) Polyostotic fibrous dysplasia
- (b) Monostotic fibrous dysplasia
- (c) Osteo-fibrous dysplasia
- (d) Parosteal osteosarcoma
- (e) Chronic osteomyelitis

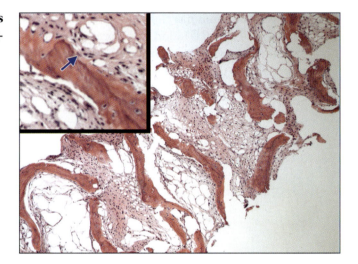

32. A 1-year-old female presents with multiple well-circumscribed nodules with the appearance seen to the right on their bilateral proximal tibia and distal femur. What germline mutation is most likely present?

- (a) P53
- (b) Rb
- (c) EXT1
- (d) PTEN
- (e) APC

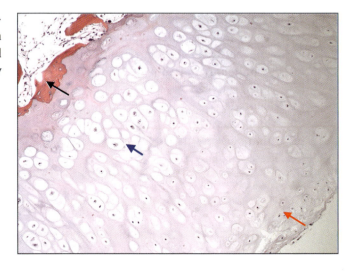

33. **A 31-year-old female has a rapidly growing right hallux well-circumscribed lesion. Histology from the lesion is shown to the right. The preoperative diagnosis was osteochondroma. What is the correct diagnosis?**
    (a) Bizarre osteochondromatous proliferation
    (b) Osteochomdroma
    (c) Solitary enchondroma
    (d) Low grade chondrosarcoma
    (e) Periosteal osteosarcoma

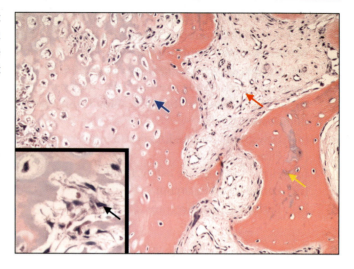

34. **A 65-year-old man has right hand numbness and a soft tissue lesion is found on ulnar nerve decompression. Histology from the lesion is shown to the right. What is the correct diagnosis?**
    (a) Enchondroma
    (b) Osteochondroma
    (c) Chondroma
    (d) Juvenile capillary hemangioma
    (e) Lobular capillary hemangioma

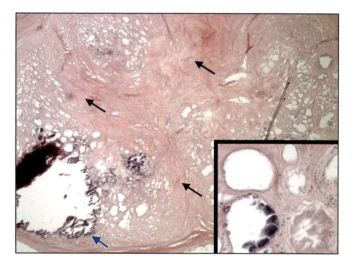

35. **This lesion is surrounded by a pseudocapsule with peripheral foci of lamellar bone. Which of the following features is least important when assessing the malignant potential of this tumor?**
    (a) Nuclear atypia
    (b) Cellularity
    (c) Mitotic activity
    (d) Infiltrative growth pattern
    (e) Presence of necrosis

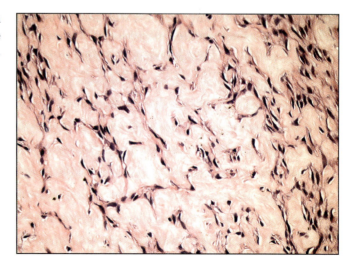

36. A 12-year-old has a lung lesion but no lesions any-where else. What is the correct diagnosis?

(a) Chondrosarcoma
(b) Extraskeletal osteosarcoma
(c) Dedifferentiated liposarcoma
(d) MPNST with heterologous differentiation
(e) Metastatic conventional osteosarcoma

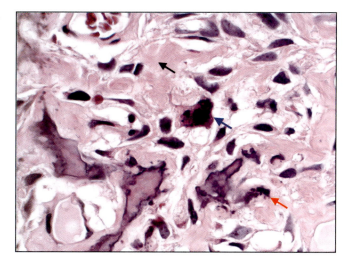

1. **(a) Conventional intramedullary osteosarcoma**

   The clinical history and histologic findings here support conventional intramedullary osteosarcoma. Most of these tumors occur in patients younger than 25 and the distal femoral metaphysis is the most common site. Histologically, a neoplastic proliferation of atypical spindled hyperchromatic cells (blue arrow) are seen with occasional woven bone production (green arrow). These cells infiltrate mature bone (red arrow). Fibrous dysplasia would feature bland spindled cells, not hyperchromatic spindled cells. Osteoid osteoma would show woven bone but would not have so prominent a spindled cell population with such atypical nuclei. Parosteal osteosarcoma features bland spindled cells and is juxtacortical. Aneurysmal bone cyst would show giant cells and woven bone with blood-filled cystic spaces and no atypia.

2. **(b) High grade surface osteosarcoma**

   This image shows atypical hyperchromatic spindled cells associated with osteoid (black arrow), consistent with high grade surface osteosarcoma or conventional osteosarcoma. Conventional osteosarcoma is histologically identical to high grade surface osteosarcoma but occurs in the medulla, not the cortex. Parosteal osteosarcoma has far less cytologic atypia than that seen here. Periosteal osteosarcoma would have more of a cartilaginous component. Desmoplastic fibroma would not feature this level of atypia, necrosis, or osteoid production.

3. **(e) Osteoblastoma**

   This is a favorable demographic for osteoblastoma, which is more common in males and usually afflicts patients between 10 and 30 years of age. Features of osteoblastoma present include contiguous regions of immature osteoid (red arrow) and osteoblast-lined (blue arrow) more mature bone (yellow arrow). Scattered osteoclast-like giant cells (black arrow) are distributed throughout this lesion and are typical for osteoblastoma. Osteoblastoma is histologically identical to osteoid osteoma but tumors greater than 2 cm are classified osteoblastoma and those smaller than 2 cm are classified osteoid osteoma. Additionally, osteoid osteoma pain would likely be relieved by aspirin but osteoblastoma pain would not. There is insufficient atypia for osteosarcoma. Giant cells are not a feature of osteofibrous or fibrous dysplasia.

4. **(c) Dedifferentiated chondrosarcoma**

   This tumor is predominantly composed of highly cellular poorly differentiated regions (black arrow and inset) which are so undifferentiated that they have lost their S-100 expression. Out of 26 sections, a 4 mm focus of well-differentiated cartilage that retained S-100 staining was seen (blue arrow). The detection of this small focus moved the diagnosis from undifferentiated sarcoma to dedifferentiated chondrosarcoma. High grade and conventional chondrosarcoma would not have well-differentiated areas abutting undifferentiated areas like seen here. Fibrosarcoma would not have chondroid regions and would have more of a fascicular pattern.

5. **(a) Low grade intramedullary chondrosarcoma**

   Low grade intramedullary chondrosarcoma most often occurs in individuals in their fourth or fifth decade of life as in this question. These lesions feature a proliferation of chondrocytes with minimal nuclear atypia (blue arrow) and minimal mitoses. Thus, enchondroma is a close differential diagnosis. The key to getting the correct diagnosis is the presence of a permeative pattern where neoplastic cartilage encircles trabecular bone (black arrow). Another diagnostic feature is the large amount of radiologic extraosseous extension by the lesion. High grade intramedullary chondrosarcoma would show higher cytologic atypia. Osteochondroma would show a cartilagenous cap with growth plate cartilagenous maturation. Enchondroma would not feature a permeative pattern and would not have the aggressive radiologic characteristics of this lesion. Chondroblastic osteosarcoma would contain osteoid, not trabecular bone.

6. **(a) Enchondroma**

   This is an enchondroma; typical features of these tumors include calcifications seen radiographically and a bluish cartilaginous matrix (blue arrow) sparsely populated by very small lacunar chondrocytes (black arrow). Cytologic atypia of these lesions is minimal except in cases of Ollier's disease or small bone enchondromas where the atypia can be mild at most. A thin bone lining can be seen with a sharp demarcation between cartilage and bone. Osteochondroma would show a cartilaginous cap over trabecular bone with histology similar to that of a normal growth plate (the hypertrophic zone would be nearest to bone which is not seen here). Low grade chondrosarcoma would show at least mild cytologic atypia or binucleation and would have a permeative appearance, not a smooth junction with bone. High grade chondrosarcoma and periosteal osteosarcoma would show cartilage with more atypia.

7. **(b) Synovial chondromatosis**
Synovial chondromatosis affects the knee in over 50% of cases. Histologically, multiple cartilaginous nodules are seen separated by thin fibrous septae (black arrow). There is mild cytologic atypia seen on the order of a low grade chondrosarcoma; however, benign radiologic features make low grade chondrosarcoma unlikely. Loose body would show some bone as well as cartilage. Chondroma occurs in small joints; a presentation in the knee would be atypical. Osteochondroma would show a cartilaginous cap mimicking a growth plate; multinodularity would not be present.

8. **(a) Ossifying fibromyxoid tumor**
Ossifying fibromyxoid tumor is characterized by cords and nests of cells deposited in a myxocollagenous matrix (black arrow). A typical finding is the presence of mature lamellar bone (blue arrow) at the periphery of the tumor and occasionally in the tumor itself, abutting the chords of tumor cells. Chondroid syringoma would have a more myxocartilagenous matrix and more complex epithelial/ myoepithelial cell architecture than what is seen here. Extraskeletal osteosarcoma would feature immature bone, not mature trabecular bone. The orbit would be an atypical site for canalicular adenoma which is usually found on the lip or palate. Retiform hemangioendothelioma would feature vascular spaces with hobnailed cells and lamellar bone would not be a part of the lesion.

9. **(b) 90%**
This is a parosteal osteosarcoma from the long tracts of bland spindled cells (black arrow) encircling woven bone (blue arrow) that is lined by osteoblasts (red arrow) and the radiologic findings of a mass wrapping around the femur. The prognosis for parosteal osteosarcoma without a dedifferentiated component is good, with a 5 year overall survival of approximately 90%. In the presence of a dedifferentiated component, the prognosis changes to that of the dedifferentiated component.

10. **(a) Metaphysis of long bones**
This is an osteochondroma characterized by a bony central region (black arrow) surrounded by a cartilaginous cap. The cartilaginous cap of osteochondroma displays epiphyseal plate maturation with hypertrophic zone chondrocytes (blue arrow) and resting zone chondrocytes (red arrow). The most common site for osteochondroma is in the metaphysis of long bones, particularly the distal femur, proximal humerus, and proximal tibia.

11. **(b) Enostosis**
This is enostosis, also known as bone island, which is an often incidentally-detected medullary bone lesion. Histologically, it is composed of lamellar bone primarily. Fracture callus would feature spindled cells and woven bone. Despite the mature, benign histologic appearance of the bone, the clinical history of a mass rules out choice C. The presence of empty lacunae raises the possibility of osteoradionecrosis; however, the patient has no significant past medical history, suggesting no history of therapeutic radiation. The most likely bone affected by osteoradionecrosis is the maxilla due to squamous cell carcinoma therapeutic radiation. Osteoblastoma would show osteoid.

12. **(b) Osteoid osteoma**
This lesion contains abundant light pink woven bone (black arrow) embedding numerous osteoblasts (red arrow), both of which are seen in osteoid osteoma. Also in osteoid osteoma the woven bone is known to entrap numerous blood vessels (blue arrow). Osteoblastoma shares similar histologic features with osteoid osteoma but by definition is greater than 2 cm. Fracture callus would show spindled cells and regenerating cartilage which are not seen. Osteosarcoma would display greater cytologic atypia and more spindled cells. Additionally, osteosarcoma usually occurs at long bones and not on the phalanges. Aneurysmal bone cyst would show blood filled spaces and giant cells which are not seen.

13. (c) Osteoma

This lesion is composed of lamellar bone. Given the lesion's location in the cortex of the ethmoid sinus, its size of 0.6 cm (most are between one half and two centimeters), and the histologic image of mature lamellar bone, the correct diagnosis is osteoma. Osteoid osteoma would show woven bone instead of lamellar bone. Bone island is a close histologic mimic; however, bone islands are medullary lesions and are not found in the cortex. Osteoradionecrosis would show some necrosis or granulation tissue. Benign bone is not consistent with the history of a lesion.

14. (d) Large cell

This is an osteosarcoma displaying prominent atypia (blue arrow) and osteoid formation (black arrow). Both skeletal and extraskeletal osteosarcomas can take on a variety of appearances including osteoblastic with atypical cells lining woven bone, chondroblastic with atypical chondrocytes and osteoid formation, small cell variant with monomorphic small round osteoid producing cells, and telangiectatic with dilated blood filled spaces lined by atypical osteoid producing cells. Large cell osteosarcoma is not a well-established subtype of osteosarcoma.

15. (c) Multiple hereditary exostoses

The lesion depicted is an osteochondroma. Histologic features include a cartilagenous cap overlying cancellous bone (black arrow). The cartilaginous cap recapitulates the layers of a growth plate including the hypertrophic zone (red arrow) and the resting zone (blue arrow). The syndrome associated with multiple osteochondromas is multiple hereditary exostoses. Gardner's syndrome is characterized by multiple osteomas. Carney complex shows pigmented skin lesions, myxomas, and endocrine abnormalities. Maffucci syndrome features multiple enchondromas. Mazabraud's syndrome includes myxomas and fibrous dysplasia.

16. (c) Telangiectatic osteosarcoma

This tumor shows large blood filled spaces (black arrow) surrounded by atypical hyperchromatic cells (red arrow) with focal light pink osteoid production (blue arrow). This triad is diagnostic of telangiectatic osteosarcoma. Angiosarcoma would show irregularly shaped spaces lined by atypical endothelial cells, not large blood filled spaces. Undifferentiated pleomorphic sarcoma and angiosarcoma would not show osteoid production. Osteosarcoma, small cell variant, shows uniform small cells with no blood filled spaces. Blood filled spaces, giant cells (yellow arrow), and osteoid can also be seen in aneurysmal bone cyst, sometimes leading to diagnostic difficulties. In general, aneurysmal bone cyst will not show the degree of cytologic atypia seen in telangiectatic osteosarcoma.

17. (b) Phosphaturic mesenchymal tumor

This image displays the classic findings of phosphaturic mesenchymal tumor, including bland spindled cells deposited in a basophilic chondromyxoid matrix (black arrow). Foci of osteoid production can be seen in these lesions (red arrow) as well as calcifications (blue arrow). Hemangiopericytoma often arises in the differential diagnosis due to the common presence of staghorn vessels (yellow arrow). Hemangiopericytoma would not feature chondromyxoid regions. Osteochondroma would have a sharp demarcation between bone and cartilage with no staghorn vessels or spindled cells. Myositis ossificans would not have basophilic matrix or staghorn vessels. Chondroblastoma shows a fibrochondroid matrix with occasional pericellular calcifications. Osteoid production and staghorn vessels are not seen in chondroblastoma.

18. (b) Spindle cell lipoma with osseous metaplasia and myxoid changes

The image depicts mature adipocytes (black arrow) intermixed with bland spindled cells (green arrow) surrounded by myxomatous and edematous regions (red arrow). Also associated with the lesion is a rim of osseous metaplasia (blue arrow). There are no hyperchromatic atypical cells present for well-differentiated liposarcoma. The cellularity and pleomorphism is too low for a dedifferentiated liposarcoma. Despite the ectopic location of bone, there is no malignant cellular proliferation associated with the lesion, making osteosarcoma unlikely. Myxoid liposarcoma would feature lipoblasts and a profoundly myxomatous stroma with a delicate vascular network which is not seen here.

19. (a) Ollier's disease

Multiple lesions are present which feature cartilage with patches of mildly increased cellularity (group of cells around black arrow) and occasionally binucleated chondrocytes (blue arrow). This low level of atypia is expected in Ollier's disease which contains multiple enchondromas with mild cytologic atypia (compared to solitary enchondroma). The atypia is not sufficient for high grade chondrosarcoma. Typical features of chondroblastoma, mononucleated cells and giant cells associated with a fibrochondroid matrix, are not seen. Chondroblastic osteosarcoma would show some osteoid production. Enchondroma is not the correct diagnosis since there are three lesions. The correct diagnosis is Ollier's disease, a disease in which patients develop multiple enchondromas. Low grade chondrosarcoma, which is not one of the answer choices, is histologically similar to an Ollier's enchondroma and would be considered if histologic bone permeation or aggressive radiologic findings were present.

20. (c) Periosteal chondroma

This periosteal chondroma shows cartilage with mildly atypical chondrocytes (blue arrow) and foci of increased cellularity (black arrow). These findings are nonspecific and can be found in enchondromas as well as low grade chondrosarcomas. The key to this diagnosis and many diagnoses in cartilage pathology is the radiologic findings. Cortical location, size smaller than 3 cm, and cortical erosion with underlying sclerosis are all features of periosteal chondroma. The relatively small size of the lesion, 1 cm, makes periosteal chondrosarcoma unlikely as most periosteal chondrosarcomas are greater than 5 cm. Enchondroma would have an intramedullary, not cortical, location. Periosteal osteosarcoma would exhibit osteoid deposition. Radiology shows a cortical, not synovial, location for this lesion, ruling out synovial chondromatosis.

21. (b) Osteoblastic osteosarcoma

Osteoblastic osteosarcoma contains highly atypical tumor cells some of which feature eosinophilic cytoplasm (red arrow) encased by immature bone (blue arrow). The immature bone displays irregular cementum lines (green arrow) in some cases of conventional osteoblastic sarcoma. Chondroblastic osteosarcoma would show chondroid differentiation at least focally. Osteosarcoma, small cell variant, would not have such large pleomorphic atypical cells. Paget's disease would show irregular cementum lines as seen but would not show the atypia seen here. Intramedullary well-differentiated osteosarcoma would not show this degree of atypia.

22. (b) Chondroblastic osteosarcoma

This is a chondromatous neoplasm (black arrow) associated with focal osteoid production (blue arrow) and a population of malignant spindled cells (red arrow), which is by definition a chondroblastic osteosarcoma. As in this case, the chondroid element can predominate but the appearance of even focal immature bone associated with tumor reclassified the tumor as a osteosarcoma. Chondrosarcoma would not show osteoid. Osteoblastic osteosarcoma would not have cartilaginous differentiation. Osteoblastoma would not have cartilage. In small cell osteosarcoma, chondroid cells do not predominate.

23. (a) Fibroblastic osteosarcoma

This lesion shows osteoid production by atypical fibroblastic cells. Fibroblastic features include atypical single stellate cells (black arrow) and fascicles of neoplastic cells reminiscent of fibrosarcoma fascicles (red arrow). A fascicular spindle cell lesion with features of malignancy that shows osteoid formation (blue arrow) is classified as a fibroblastic osteosarcoma. Chondroblastic osteosarcoma would show some chondroid differentiation. Osteoid osteoma and osteoblastoma are benign entities that are not consistent with the radiologically necrotic and invasive nature of the lesion. Furthermore, these lesions would not have such atypical cells. Fibrosarcoma would not show osteoid.

24. (e) Reactive osteochondromatous proliferation

This lesion has several features that can be found in reactive osteochondromatous proliferations such as Nora's lesion and fibro-osseous pseudotumor of digits, including osteoblastic rimming (black arrow), woven bone (blue arrow), cartilaginous differentiation (red arrow), and an intermingled population of bland plump myofibroblasts (green arrow). Imaging studies show these lesions to be localized to the soft tissue and occasionally involve the periosteum. Despite the osteoblastic rimming and woven bone, cartilaginous differentiation and a myofibroblastic population are not consistent with osteoid osteoma. There are no chicken wire calcifications that can be seen in chondroblastoma and osteoid deposition is not a feature of chondroblastoma. Osteochondroma would not show osteoblastic rimming. Fibrous dysplasia would not feature chondroid differentiation.

25. **(b) Giant cell reparative granuloma**

    This lesion shows sparsely distributed giant cells surrounded by hemorrhage (black arrow), bland fibroblasts (red arrow), and focal osteoid production (blue arrow), all features that are consistent with giant cell reparative granuloma. Giant cells are not seen prominently in fracture callus. Well-differentiated intramedullary osteosarcoma would show more atypia. Nonossifying fibroma shares several common features with giant cell reparative granuloma but it would not show osteoid production. Giant cell tumor of tendon sheath does not typically have osteoid and is not a bone tumor.

26. **(a) Amplification of 12q13-15**

    The clinical history is indicative of parosteal osteosarcoma since it is a patient in their third decade with a mass wrapping around the posterior aspect of the tibia (proximal tibia and distal femur are favored). Additionally, the fact that the lesion has been present for some time suggests the indolent nature of parosteal osteosarcoma. Histologically, long fascicular tracts of bland spindled cells (black arrow) associated with woven bone (red arrow) and osteoblastic rimming (blue arrow) are seen, all features of parosteal osteosarcoma. Chromosomal region 12q13-15 is amplified in most parosteal osteosarcoma cases. 17p13 translocations are found in aneurysmal bone cysts but aneurysmal bone cyst would show blood filled spaces accompanying woven bone and giant cells. T(11;22) translocations are seen in Ewing's sarcoma. T(12;15) translocations are seen in congenital fibrosarcoma. T(12;22) is seen in clear cell sarcoma. None of these three sarcomas should show woven bone with osteoblastic rimming.

27. **(a) Myositis ossificans**

    This lesion has several features of myositis ossificans including a central granulation tissue-type area with sparsely distributed spindled and stellate cells (yellow arrow) and chondroid regions (black arrow) abutting areas of osteoid deposition (blue arrow). Lastly, a rim of fibroblasts is seen surrounding and intermixing with the osteoid (red arrow). Not seen here is the most peripheral portion of most cases of myositis ossificans, a rim of mature lamellar bone, which creates the characteristic "zoning pattern". There is not enough atypia for extraskeletal osteosarcoma. Chondrosarcoma would not feature central granulation tissue-type areas and osteoid. Fibrosarcoma would be more cellular with a herringbone pattern with no osteoid formation. Nodular fasciitis would not explain the bone and cartilage.

28. **(d) Chondroid lipoma**

    Chondroid lipoma, also known as lipoma with chondroid changes, displays hyalinized nodules (blue arrow) deposited in mature adipose tissue (black arrow). The nodules can show chondroid differentiation occasionally. The other answer choices do not feature hyalinized nodules.

29. **(c) Osteochondroma**

    The history of pain for some time and a mass with no soft tissue invasion is suggestive of osteochondroma. Microscopically, we see the diagnostic hallmarks of osteochondroma: A bony stalk (black arrow) over which a thin cartilaginous cap grows. The cap recapitulates the physiologic layers of a benign epiphyseal plate including the hypertrophic zone (blue arrow) and the resting zone (red arrow). Parosteal osteosarcoma would feature a spindled cell component. Chondrosarcoma can have a benign histologic appearance; however, some radiologic or histologic evidence of invasion should be present. Osteoid osteoma is a well-circumscribed bone forming lesion and lacks a cartilaginous component. Osteopetrosis would not appear as a mass with cartilaginous maturation.

30. **(a) Low grade intramedullary osteosarcoma**

    This histology shows fascicles of bland spindled cells (black arrow) growing around trabecular bone. The lack of cytologic atypia rules out high grade surface osteosarcoma. The lack of cartilage rules out periosteal osteosarcoma. Fibrous dysplasia, parosteal osteosarcoma, and low grade intramedulllary osteosarcoma have a similar histologic appearance and require radiology to distinguish them. Radiologically, fibrous dysplasia is medullary based like low grade intramedullary osteosarcoma but it is well-circumscribed with minimal periosteal reaction, in contrast to the aggressive lesion described here. Parosteal osteosarcoma is centered on the cortical surface, not in the medulla.

31. (a) Polyostotic fibrous dysplasia

The lesion shows the characteristic curvilinear bony trabeculae of fibrous dysplasia separated by bland fibrous spindled cells. Osteo-fibrous dysplasia is a close differential; however, the trabecular surface only shows bland fibrous cells (blue arrow) and not osteoblastic rimming, ruling out osteo-fibrous dysplasia. Furthermore, osteo-fibrous dysplasia is a cortical not a medullary lesion. In the question stem, there are multiple lesions; thus monostotic fibrous dysplasia is not correct. Biopsies of a parosteal osteosarcoma may enter the differential diagnosis with fibrous dysplasia but parosteal osteosarcoma is rarely found in the medulla of the bone and the cells show at least mild atypia, always absent in fibrous dysplasia. Fibrosis can be associated with chronic osteomyelitis but the hallmark of chronic osteomyelitis, the plasma cell, is not present.

32. (c) EXT1

This is an osteochondroma featuring a bony stalk (black arrow) with a thin cartilaginous cap. The cap displays normal epiphyseal plate maturation with a hypertrophic zone (blue arrow) and a resting zone (red arrow). Multiple osteochondromas (hereditary multiple exostoses) is an autosomal dominant disease caused by mutations in the tumor suppressor genes EXT1 or EXT2 predominantly. The remaining answer choices are tumor suppressor genes not associated with osteochondromas.

33. (a) Bizarre osteochondromatous proliferation

The age range is correct for bizarre osteochondromatous proliferation (Nora's lesion) since Nora's lesions typically occurs in patients between 20 and 40 years of age. Preferred sites include the hand and feet bones as in this case and the well-circumscribed radiologic appearance is consistent with osteochondroma or Nora's lesion. Histologically, this lesion is composed of areas which are more chondroid and areas that are made up of bone (yellow arrow) with interspersed anastomosing bland fibrous islands (red arrow), all of which are characteristic of Nora's lesion. Irregular transitions from cartilage to bone also support the diagnosis of Nora's lesion (blue arrow). The fibrous islands, irregular osteochondromatous transitions, and mild to moderate chondrocytic atypia with hypercellularity (black arrow) seen in this case rule out osteochondroma. Solitary enchondroma would have less atypia and osseous regions with irregular transitions are not consistent with enchondroma. Low grade chondrosarcoma would show aggressive radiologic characteristics with a permeative involvement of bone that is not seen here. Periosteal osteosarcoma prefers long bones such as the femur, tibia, and humerus.

34. (c) Chondroma

In chondroma, thick fibrous septae (black arrows) separate lobules of cartilage. In some cases, the cartilage undergoes calcific changes, leading to total replacement of the cartilage with calcified spaces (blue arrow and inset). Thick fibrous septae are not seen in enchondroma or osteochondroma. Lobular capillary hemangioma and juvenile capillary hemangioma show thick fibrous septae but would display a vascular component.

35. (e) Presence of necrosis

This tumor is an ossifying fibromyxoid tumor, identified by cords of bland spindled cells deposited in a myxocollagenous matrix. These tumors also contain a peripheral rim of lamellar bone surrounding the lesion as described in the question stem. Features most associated with malignant behavior include nuclear atypia, high cellularity, and increased mitotic activity. An infiltrative growth pattern has also been associated with an increased chance of recurrence.

36. (b) Extraskeletal osteosarcoma

This tumor shows osteoid (black arrow), mitoses (red arrow), and highly atypical cells (blue arrow), all consistent with osteosarcoma. The absence of lesions outside the lung, specifically in the bone, rules out metastatic conventional osteosarcoma. The presence of osteoid rules out chondrosarcoma. Dedifferentiated liposarcoma would be a diagnostic consideration if the patient had a retroperitoneal mass; however, extraskeletal osteosarcoma is more likely with a solitary lung lesion. MPNST would be a consideration if the patient had a history of neurofibromatosis.

INDEX

Page numbers followed by *f* and *t* refer to figures and tables respectively.

A

Adamantinoma 114
Adenomatous polyposis coli 60
Adult rhabdomyoma 102
Alveolar rhabdomyosarcoma 125, 126
Ancient schwannoma 23
Aneurysmal bone cyst 114
Angiofibroma 74
Angioleiomyoma 75
Angiolipoma 73, 116
Angiomatoid fibrous histiocytoma 106
Angiomatosis 74, 76
Angiomyofibroblastoma 27
Angiomyolipoma 76
Angiomyxoma, aggressive 87
Angiosarcoma 143
Aponeurotic fibroma 25
Atypical fibroxanthoma 46

B

Bacillary angiomatosis 73
Baker's cyst 114, 115
Bizarre osteochondromatous
        proliferation 151
Brown tumor 114

C

Calcifying fibrous tumor 103
Campanacci's disease 115
Cavernous hemangioma 74
Cellular schwannoma 25
Chondroblastic osteosarcoma 149
Chondroblastoma 116, 148
Chondroid lipoma 150
Chondroid syringoma 147
Chondroma 151
Chondromyxoid fibroma 85
Chondrosarcoma 146, 150
Chordoma 105
Clear cell chondrosarcoma 132
Clear cell sarcoma 103

Conventional intramedullary
        chondrosarcoma 87
Conventional intramedullary
        osteosarcoma 146
Cutaneous angiomyxoma 86

D

Dermal nerve sheath myxoma 85
Dermatofibroma 25
Dermatofibrosarcoma protuberans 10, 25
Desmoid fibromatosis 24, 31
Desmoplastic fibroblastoma 30
Desmoplastic fibroma 24
Desmoplastic small round blue
        cell tumor 124
Dupuytren's contracture 27, 31

E

Edward's syndrome 75
Elastofibroma 30
Embryonal rhabdomyosarcoma 28, 126
Enchondroma 141, 146
Enostosis 147
Epithelioid hemangioendothelioma 75
Epithelioid hemangioma 73, 76
Epithelioid sarcoma 103
Erlenmeyer flask deformity 95
Ewing's sarcoma 116, 125
Extraskeletal myxoid chondrosarcoma 87
Extraskeletal osteosarcoma 147, 151

F

Familial adenomatous polyposis
        syndrome 31
Fetal rhabdomyoma 29
Fibroblastic osteosarcoma 149
Fibroma of tendon sheath 30
Fibro-osseous pseudotumor 30
Fibrosarcoma 31
        high grade 48
Fibrous dysplasia 150
Fibrous hamartoma of infancy 27

G

Ganglion cyst 83, 114, 115
Ganglioneuroblastoma 27, 124
Ganglioneuroma 23
Gardner's syndrome 148
Gaucher disease 104
Giant cell fibroblastoma 46
Giant cell reparative granuloma 150
Glomus tumor 105
Gout 60
Granular cell tumor 104
Granuloma annulare 100

H

Hemosiderotic synovitis 116
Hibernoma 102
Hodgkin's lymphoma 46, 114

I

Infantile digital fibroma 23
Infantile fibromatosis 31
Infantile fibrosarcoma 27
Inflammatory myofibroblastic tumor 24
Intestinal lipomatosis 60
Intramuscular myxoma 88
Ischemic fasciitis 28

J

Jaffe-Campanacci syndrome 131
Juvenile capillary hemangioma 76
Juvenile hyaline fibromatosis 25
Juvenile xanthogranuloma 102
Juxta-articular myxoma 88

K

Kaposi's sarcoma 73, 75
Kaposiform hemangioendothelioma 74
Kasabach-Merritt syndrome 75
Kimura's disease 76

L

Langerhans cell histiocytosis 114, 116

Leiomyoma of deep soft tissue 30
Leiomyosarcoma 50
Liposarcoma 46, 47, 49
Lobular capillary hemangioma 65
Low-grade
    fibromyxosarcoma 88
    intramedullary
        chondrosarcoma 146
        osteosarcoma 150
    myxofibrosarcoma 86
Lymphangioma 75
Lymphangiomatosis 74

M

Maffucci syndrome 148
Malignant extrarenal rhabdoid tumor 102
Malignant peripheral nerve sheath
    tumor 48, 51
Malignant tenosynovial giant cell
    tumor 131
Mazabraud's syndrome 148
McCune-Albright syndrome 116
Medulloblastoma 125
Melanotic neuroectodermal tumor 125
Melanotic schwannoma 29
Mesenchymal chondrosarcoma 126
Monostotic fibrous dysplasia 28
Multiple hereditary exostoses 148
Myelolipoma 59
Myoepithelioma 105
Myofibroblastic sarcoma, high-grade 49
Myofibroblastoma 25
Myofibroma 23, 30
Myofibromatosis 26
Myolipoma 30
Myopericytoma 76
Myositis ossificans 150
Myxofibrosarcoma, high-grade 86
Myxoid chondrosarcoma 126
Myxoid liposarcoma 75, 84, 85, 87, 102
Myxoid neurothekeoma 86
Myxoinflammatory fibroblastic
    sarcoma 50

N

Necrotizing fasciitis 60

Neuroblastoma 125
Neurofibroma 26
Neuroma 27
Neurothekeoma 28
Niemann-Pick Disease 104
Nodular fasciitis 24
Nodular Kaposi sarcoma 23
Nonossifying fibroma 107, 115
Nora's lesion 151
Nuchal type fibroma 59

O

Odontogenic myxoma 86
Ollier's disease 147, 148
Ossifying fibroma 107
Ossifying fibromyxoid tumor 147
Osteoarthritis 60
Osteoblastic osteosarcoma 149
Osteoblastoma 146
Osteochondroma 144, 150
Osteofibrous dysplasia 114
Osteoid osteoma 147
Osteoma 148
Osteomalacia 75
Osteomyelitis
    acute 59
    chronic 59
Osteopenia 59
Osteopetrosis 59

P

Paget's disease of bone 115
Papillary endothelial hyperplasia 76
Paraganglioma 106
Parosteal osteosarcoma 31, 150
Patch-stage Kaposi sarcoma 23
Perineurioma 28
Phosphaturic mesenchymal tumor 148
Plasma cell neoplasm 115
Pleomorphic lipoma 51
Pleomorphic liposarcoma 46
Pleomorphic rhabdomyosarcoma 105
Plexiform fibrohistiocytic tumor 103

Polyostotic fibrous dysplasia 116, 151
Proliferative myositis 26
Pyogenic granuloma 73

R

Retiform hemangioendothelioma 147
Retinoblastoma 124
Rhabdomyosarcoma 108
Rheumatoid arthritis 60
Round cell liposarcoma 86

S

Sclerosing epithelioid fibrosarcoma 105
Septic arthritis 60
Sheehan's syndrome 75
Solitary fibrous tumor 29
Spindle cell
    hemangioma 73
    lipoma 29, 116, 139, 148
Superficial acral fibromyxoma 85
Synovial chondromatosis 147
Synovial hemangioma 74
Synovial lipomatosis 116
Synovial sarcoma 51

T

Telangiectatic osteosarcoma 148
Tenosynovial giant cell tumor 131
Terminal osseous dysplasia 29
Traumatic neuroma 26
Tuberous sclerosis 30
Tuberous xanthoma 104

U

Unicameral bone cysts 115

W

Wilms' tumor 126

X

Xanthoma 102

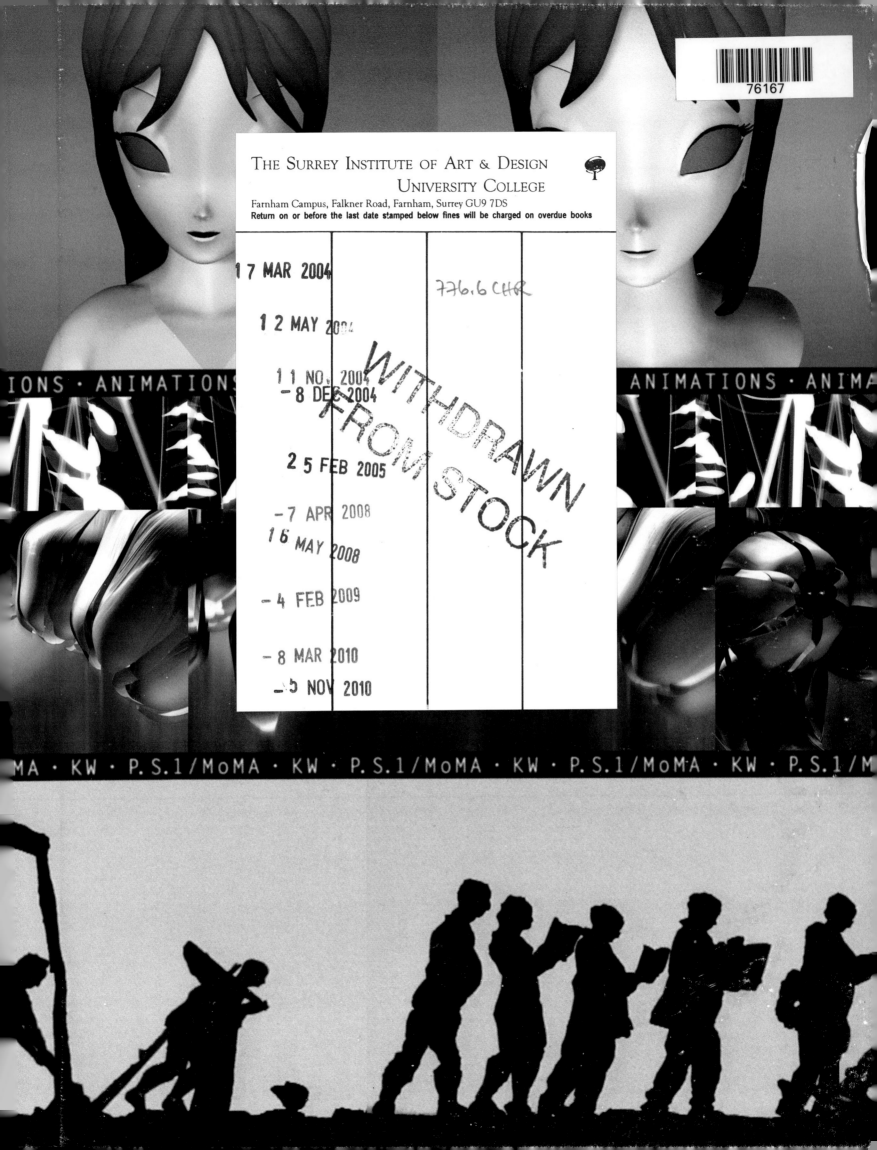